THE PULSE OF PROGRESS

Stuart Pharmaceuticals is deeply committed to discovery.

The pulse of our research efforts is targeted against the intractable diseases of our time... *particularly in the cardiovascular area.* And our commitment is enhanced by our affiliation with the extensive research of ICI Pharmaceuticals in England. That research has led to the development and introduction worldwide of:

- the first beta blocker
- the first specific antilipidemic agent
- the world's most widely used antimicrobial skin cleanser
- a non-steroidal antiestrogen that offers breast cancer patients a better quality of life.

Stuart's commitment continues... with a pledge to both you and your patients. *To maintain the pulse that carries research to realization.*

STUART PHARMACEUTICALS | Div. of ICI Americas Inc.
WILMINGTON, DELAWARE 19897

self-assessment of current knowledge in
Internal Medicine
fourth edition

583 multiple choice questions and referenced answers

Edited by

JAMES W. HOLSINGER, Jr., M.D., Ph.D.
Chief of Staff
Veterans Administration Medical Center
Professor of Medicine and Anatomy
Medical College of Georgia
Augusta, Georgia

Medical Examination Publishing Co., Inc.
an Excerpta Medica company

969 Stewart Avenue • Garden City, New York 11530

Copyright © 1980 by
MEDICAL EXAMINATION
PUBLISHING CO., INC.
an *Excerpta Medica* company

Library of Congress Card Number
79-91971

ISBN   0-87488-257-5

January, 1980

All rights reserved. No part of this
publication may be reproduced in any
form or by any means, electronic or
mechanical, including photocopy,
without permission in writing from
the publisher.

Printed in the United States of America

preface

The authors have prepared this book for the purpose of assisting those individuals who wish to assess their current knowledge in Internal Medicine. It should allow the individual to assess his strengths and weaknesses, as well as stimulate him to comprehensively review the subject.

The book is divided into several sections pertaining to the various recognized subspecialties in the field of Internal Medicine. As such, each section can be utilized as a method for briefly reviewing the current status of each subspecialty. In addition, by utilizing all sections an assessment of current knowledge in Internal Medicine may be obtained.

The types of questions offered in this text were prepared utilizing standard board examination formats. However, it should be remembered that although the questions have been written based upon important articles or recent texts, the ability to choose the correct answer is not as important as having read, studied, and assimilated the material.

James W. Holsinger, Jr., M.D., Ph.D.
Editor

contributors

SAMIR K. BALLAS, M.D., *Assistant Professor of Medicine,* Jefferson Medical College, Thomas Jefferson University, Philadelphia, Pennsylvania

JOHN F. FOLEY, M.D., *Professor of Medicine,* Division of Oncology, Department of Internal Medicine, The University of Nebraska Medical Center, Omaha, Nebraska

ARMIN F. HAERER, M.D., *Professor of Neurology,* The University of Mississippi Medical Center, School of Medicine, Jackson, Mississippi

JAMES W. HOLSINGER, Jr., M.D., Ph.D., *Chief of Staff,* Veterans Administration Medical Center; *Professor of Medicine and Anatomy,* Medical College of Georgia, Augusta, Georgia

WILLIAM K.C. MORGAN, M.D., *Director,* Sir Adam Beck Chest Unit; *Professor of Medicine,* University of Western Ontario, London, Ontario, Canada

DAVID A. ONTJES, M.D., *Professor of Medicine and Pharmacology; Chief,* Endocrine Division, Division of Health Affairs, Department of Medicine, The University of North Carolina at Chapel Hill, Chapel Hill, North Carolina

ROBERT E. PIERONI, M.D., F.A.A.F.P., *Associate Professor of Internal Medicine; Associate Professor of Family Medicine,* College of Community Health Sciences, The University of Alabama, University, Alabama

MARTIN J. RAFF, M.D., *Associate Chairman,* Department of Medicine (Clinical Service); *Associate Professor of Medicine; Chief,* Section of Infectious Disease, Department of Medicine, University of Louisville School of Medicine; *Associate Chief of Staff,* University Hospital, Louisville, Kentucky

EARL C. SMITH, M.D., *Associate Professor of Medicine,* Rush Medical College of Rush University; *Chief,* Nephrology Division, Mount Sinai Hospital, Medical Center of Chicago, Chicago, Illinois

WILLIAM A. SODEMAN, Jr., M.D., *Professor and Chairman,* Department of Comprehensive Medicine, University of South Florida Medical Center, College of Medicine, Tampa, Florida

contents

   I Cardiology 1

  II Hematology 27

 III Neurology 41

 IV Infectious Diseases 50

  V Endocrinology 77

 VI Rheumatology 113

VII Nephrology 131

VIII Gastroenterology 151

 IX Pulmonary 173

  X Oncology 192

      Answers and Comments 202

notice

The editor and publisher of this book have made every effort to ensure that all therapeutic modalities that are recommended are in accordance with accepted standards at the time of publication.

The drugs specified within this book may not have specific approval by the Food and Drug Administration in regard to the indications and dosages that are recommended by the editor. The manufacturer's package insert is the best source of current prescribing information.

Questions

I: Cardiology

DIRECTIONS: Each of the questions or incomplete statements below is followed by four or five suggested answers or completions. Select the **one** that is **BEST** in each case.

1. Which of the following is the most common cause of nonrheumatic mitral regurgitation?
   A. mitral valve prolapse
   B. postinfarction mitral regurgitation
   C. isolated rupture of chordae tendineae
   D. congenital mitral regurgitation
   E. postendocarditic mitral regurgitation
   REF: Mod. Concepts Cardiovasc. Dis. 48:25-30, 1979

2. The major indication for coronary artery bypass surgery is
   A. crescendo angina
   B. to lower mortality
   C. left main coronary artery disease
   D. relief of angina pectoris
   REF: N. Engl. J. Med. 300:149-157, 1979

2 / Cardiology

3. Which of the following disorders is most commonly found as an antecedent to the development of left bundle branch block (LBBB)?
   A. diabetes
   B. coronary heart disease
   C. hypertension
   D. cardiac enlargement seen on chest x-ray
   E. congestive heart disease
   REF: Ann. Intern. Med. 90:303-310, 1979

4. The most common side effect of β-blocking drugs is
   A. congestive heart failure
   B. impotence
   C. hallucinations
   D. bronchoconstriction
   REF: Curr. Probl. Cardiol. 3 (No. 10):1-53, 1979

5. In the treatment of hypertension, the side effects of prazosin are caused by
   A. β-blockade
   B. direct vasodilation
   C. postsynaptic α-adrenoreceptor blockade
   D. presynaptic α-adrenoreceptor blockade
   REF: Ibid.

6. Which of the following is NOT a synonym for unstable angina pectoris?
   A. preinfarction angina
   B. intermediate syndrome
   C. coronary insufficiency
   D. unstable angina
   E. all of the above
   REF: Bristow, J.W.: A cardiologist's view of coronary bypass surgery. In: Yu, P.N. and Goodwin, J.F., *Progress in Cardiology, Vol. 6*, Lea & Febiger, Philadelphia, 1977, pp. 1-40

7. The average incidence of perioperative myocardial infarction associated with coronary artery bypass surgery is
   A. 0%–2%
   B. 5%–10%
   C. 10%–15%
   D. 15%–20%
   REF: Ibid.

8. Which of the following is NOT an indication for treatment of ventricular premature complexes?
   A. primary ventricular fibrillation unprovoked by acute myocardial infarction (MI)
   B. arrhythmia without severe symptoms
   C. advanced grade of ventricular premature complexes during angina pectoris
   D. coronary artery disease and ventricular tachycardia during the vulnerable period of monitoring
   REF: Am. J. Cardiol. 43:313-328, 1979

9. Which of the following is NOT a radionuclide indicator available for assessment of regional myocardial perfusion?
   A. mercurial compounds
   B. potassium analogues (Thallium - 201)
   C. particulate indicators
   D. diffusible inert gases (Xenon-133)
   REF: Am. Heart J. 97:112-118, 1979

10. Which of the following currently available cationic tracers is the best for myocardial perfusion imaging?
    A. potassium-43
    B. cesium-129
    C. rubidium-81
    D. thallium-201
    REF: Ibid.

11. Which portion of the heart is visualized in the normal myocardial perfusion scan?
    A. left ventricle
    B. right ventricle
    C. left atrium
    D. right atrium
    REF: Ibid.

12. For lesions in the myocardium to be considered significant on a myocardial perfusion scan, their radioactivity must vary from adjacent areas by
    A. 10%
    B. 20%
    C. 30%
    D. 40%
    REF: Ibid.

13. Which of the following is the treatment of choice for hypercholesterolemia?
    A. exercise
    B. nicotinic acid
    C. diet
    D. clofibrate
    REF: Am. Heart J. 97:389-398, 1979

14. The optimal level of serum cholesterol for retardation of atherosclerosis may be under
    A. 170 mg/dl
    B. 200 mg/dl
    C. 240 mg/dl
    D. 300 mg/dl
    REF: Ibid.

15. Of the following cholesterol-lowering drugs, which is the most potent?
    A. clofibrate
    B. dextrothyroxine
    C. nicotinic acid
    D. bile acid-binding resins
    REF: Ibid.

16. Following the administration of systemic vasodilators, stroke volume increases owing to a transient
    A. increase in cardiac output
    B. reduction in arterial pressure
    C. decrease in systemic resistance
    D. increase in systemic vasodilation
    REF: Am. Heart J. 97:519-526, 1979

17. Which of the following is NOT a physiologic determinant of myocardial oxygen demand?
    A. coronary blood flow
    B. left ventricular wall tension
    C. myocardial contractility
    D. heart rate
    REF: Am. Heart J. 97:527-534, 1979

18. Which of the following is NOT characteristic of cardiac myxoma?
    A. occurs predominantly in women
    B. usually occurs in the left atrium
    C. age 27 ± 5 years
    D. duration of symptoms averages 15 months
    REF: Am. Heart J. 97:639-643, 1979

19. Which of the following is the most common clinical sign or symptom of myxoma?
    A. pulmonary edema
    B. chest pain
    C. mitral stenosis murmur
    D. congestive heart failure
    REF: Ibid.

20. Which of the following inhibitors of glycolysis produces a reduction of the action potential duration?
    A. iodoacetate
    B. high pH
    C. lactate
    D. pyruvate
    REF: Am. J. Cardiol. 43:131-148, 1979

21. Which of the following is the most common symptom of constrictive pericarditis?
    A. abdominal distention
    B. peripheral edema
    C. dyspnea
    D. orthopnea
    REF: Am. Heart J. 96:110-122, 1978

22. Which of the following is the most common physical sign associated with constrictive pericarditis?
    A. ascites
    B. distended neck veins
    C. hepatomegaly
    D. peripheral edema
    REF: Ibid.

23. The treatment of choice for pericardial constriction is
    A. vigorous diuretic therapy
    B. paracentesis
    C. pericardiectomy
    D. digitalis
    REF: Ibid.

24. Which of the following diagnostic techniques is the most definitive in infective endocarditis?
    A. echocardiography
    B. cardiac catheterization
    C. serologic test
    D. blood culture
    REF: Am. Heart J. 96:123-128, 1978

25. In patients with suspected infective endocarditis, when should blood cultures be obtained?
    A. one to three cultures as soon as infective endocarditis suspected
    B. three to six cultures over a period of hours to days
    C. six cultures each time the patient spikes a fever
    D. six cultures each day for five days
    REF: Ibid.

26. In what percentage of patients with infective endocarditis of six weeks or more duration will rheumatoid factor in blood be found?
    A. 20%
    B. 50%
    C. 67%
    D. 80%
    REF: Ibid.

27. Which of the following organisms is usually associated with bacteremias following dental procedures?
    A. *Staphylococcus aureus*
    B. *Pseudomonas aeruginosa*
    C. *Streptococcus bovis*
    D. *S. viridans*
    REF: Am. Heart J. 96:263-269, 1978

28. Which of the following is NOT a hazard in the use of intravenous nitroglycerin?
    A. decreased coronary artery perfusion pressure
    B. tachycardia
    C. decreased myocardial oxygen demand
    D. intramyocardial steal syndrome
    REF: Am. Heart J. 96:550-553, 1978

29. Which of the following is NOT an absolute contraindication to exercise testing?
    A. recent myocardial infarction
    B. unstable angina pectoris with recent episodes of rest pain
    C. overt congestive heart failure
    D. serious ventricular arrhythmia at rest
    REF: Am. Heart J. 95:102-114, 1978

30. Which of the following is an absolute indication for early termination of an exercise test?
    A. cyanosis or pallor
    B. chest pain
    C. excessive ST-segment depression
    D. frequent ventricular premature beats including bigeminy and multifocal ectopy
    REF: Ibid.

31. Which of the following is NOT descriptive of prazosin?
    A. potent inhibitor of cyclic AMP hydrolysis
    B. slowly absorbed by various tissues
    C. plasma half-life of one to two hours
    D. excreted in stool and urine
    REF: Am. Heart J. 95:262-265, 1978

32. Which of the following adverse effects of prazosin is most troublesome?
    A. dizziness
    B. fatigue and weakness
    C. palpitations
    D. first-dose phenomenon
    REF: Ibid.

33. Total plasma creatine kinase following the onset of chest pain in acute myocardial infarction peaks within
    A. 4 to 8 hours
    B. 12 to 24 hours
    C. 36 to 48 hours
    D. 72 to 96 hours
    REF: Am. Heart J. 95:521-528, 1978

34. Which isoenzyme of creatine kinase is virtually specific for myocardial injury?
    A. MM
    B. BB
    C. MB
    REF: Ibid.

35. Creatine kinase is present in the largest concentration in which of the following tissues?
    A. kidney
    B. brain
    C. muscle
    D. heart
    REF: Ibid.

36. Which of the following vasopressors has the most prompt and potent actions in the patient in shock following acute MI?
    A. norepinephrine
    B. dopamine
    C. metaraminol
    D. epinephrine
    REF: Am. Heart J. 95:529-534, 1978

37. In the shock state associated with acute myocardial infarction the cardiac index is usually less than
    A. 3.0 L/min/m²
    B. 2.3 L/min/m²
    C. 1.8 L/min/m²
    D. 1.5 L/min/m²
    REF: Ibid.

38. Which of the following statements concerning magnesium is NOT true?
    A. magnesium in large concentration has a curariform action on the neuromuscular junction
    B. severe magnesium deficiency is manifested by hyperexcitability and occasional behavioral disturbances
    C. magnesium increases blood lipids
    D. magnesium decreases blood coagulability
    REF: Am. Heart J. 94:649-657, 1977

39. Which of the following cations is the most plentiful in the human body?
    A. magnesium
    B. potassium
    C. sodium
    D. calcium
    REF: Ibid.

40. Which of the following is NOT consistent with bacterial shock?
    A. increased serum transaminase
    B. decreased serum amylase
    C. leukopenia and thrombocytopenia followed by leukocytosis
    D. ST-segment and T-wave abnormalities on ECG
    REF: Am. Heart J. 94:112-114, 1977

41. If dopamine is used in the treatment of bacterial shock, the arterial pressure for the individual patient should be maintained at
    A. 20-30 mm Hg above normal
    B. normal
    C. 10-15 mm Hg below normal
    D. 20-30 mm Hg below normal
    REF: Ibid.

42. On the basis of echocardiographic criteria, the incidence of mitral valve prolapse has been reported to be
    A. 1%-2%
    B. 3%-6%
    C. 6%-12%
    D. 12%-20%
    REF: Am. Heart J. 94:227-249, 1977

43. On echocardiogram which of the following may be mistaken for pericardial effusion?
    A. constrictive pericarditis
    B. dilated left atrium
    C. left pleural effusion
    D. atrial septal defect
    REF: Ibid.

Cardiology / 11

44. Which of the following symptoms of cardiac pacemaker malfunction may indicate the loss of adequate sensing and competitive pacer rhythms?
   A. syncope
   B. palpitations
   C. rhythmic waves of weakness
   D. return of original symptoms
   REF: Am. Heart J. 94:378-386, 1977

45. Which of the following is NOT a change noted in saphenous vein used as aortocoronary bypass grafts?
   A. endothelial damage
   B. medial hypertrophy
   C. medial necrosis
   D. adventitial thinning
   REF: Am. Heart J. 94:500-516, 1977

46. Which of the following is NOT a factor that promotes fibrinous or fibrous intimal proliferation in saphenous veins used for aortocoronary bypass grafts?
   A. ninety degree angle of aortic anastomosis
   B. severe narrowing distal to graft insertion
   C. insertion of graft in area of plaque
   D. tension on grafted vein
   REF: Ibid.

47. Which of the following objective findings is most common in adult patients with discrete subaortic stenosis?
   A. cardiomegaly
   B. systolic murmur
   C. left ventricular hypertrophy
   D. pressure gradient from left ventricle to aorta
   REF: Am. J. Cardiol. 42:283-290, 1978

48. Which of the following is the most common clinical finding in adult patients with discrete subaortic stenosis?
    A. chest pain
    B. palpitations
    C. fatigue
    D. exertional dyspnea
    REF: Ibid.

49. The most common cardiac lesion associated with discrete subaortic stenosis is
    A. congenital aortic valve stenosis
    B. supravalvular obstruction
    C. acquired aortic insufficiency
    D. rheumatic valvular heart disease
    REF: Ibid.

50. What percent of patients with hypertrophic obstructive cardiomyopathy are found to have life-threatening arrhythmias?
    A. 10%
    B. 20%
    C. 35%
    D. 50%
    REF: Am. J. Cardiol. 42:993-1001, 1978

51. What is the effective dose of propranolol that should be used in the long-term medical management of hypertrophic obstructive cardiomyopathy?
    A. 120 mg/day
    B. 320 mg/day
    C. 480 mg/day
    D. 720 mg/day
    REF: Ibid.

52. Which type of tachycardia is most suitable for treatment with temporary electrical pacing?
    A. atrial fibrillation
    B. atrial flutter
    C. junctional tachycardia
    D. ventricular flutter
    REF: Am. J. Cardiol. 41:1025-1034, 1978

53. In patients with preexcitation and a short refractory period of the accessory pathway, rapid atrial pacing may induce
    A. sinus tachycardia
    B. atrial flutter
    C. atrial fibrillation
    D. junctional tachycardia
    REF: Ibid.

54. What percent of patients admitted to the hospital with anginal pain have "variant" angina?
    A. 2%
    B. 5%
    C. 10%
    D. 20%
    REF: Am. J. Cardiol. 42:1019-1035, 1978

55. Which of the following diagnostic procedures is useful in establishing the diagnosis of "variant" angina?
    A. thallium-201 myocardial scan during angina at rest
    B. continuous hemodynamic monitoring
    C. exercise stress testing
    D. echocardiography
    REF: Ibid.

DIRECTIONS: For each of the following questions or incomplete statements, **ONE** or **MORE** of the answers or completions given is correct. Select:
  A if only 1, 2 and 3 are correct,
  B if only 1 and 3 are correct,
  C if only 2 and 4 are correct,
  D if only 4 is correct,
  E if all are correct.

56. Papillary muscle rupture in acute myocardial infarction
    1. carries a mortality of 80%-90%
    2. produces a treatable form of cardiogenic shock
    3. is not associated with a critical mass of myocardial injury
    4. damages at least 40% of the left ventricular mass
    REF: Ann. Intern. Med. 90:149-153, 1979

57. The treatment of choice for idiopathic mitral valve prolapse is
    1. mitral valve replacement aimed at the elimination of arrhythmias
    2. aggressive treatment of all patients with arrhythmias
    3. surgical mitral valve replacement following cardiac catheterization for patients with cardiac failure
    4. treatment of asymptomatic patients with standard protective measures against endocarditis
    REF: Mod. Concepts Cardiovasc. Dis. 48:25-30, 1979

58. Which of the following indicators is (are) among the most characteristic traits of the youthful coronary patient?
    1. restlessness during leisure hours
    2. high resting heart rate
    3. sense of guilt during periods of relaxation
    4. increased speed of reaction
    REF: Mod. Concepts Cardiovasc. Dis. 48:19-24, 1979

59. Compared with medical treatment, the results of coronary artery bypass for stable angina demonstrate
    1. greater functional improvement
    2. unchanged likelihood of death
    3. less unstable angina
    4. unchanged likelihood of myocardial infarction
    REF: N. Engl. J. Med. 300:149-157, 1979

60. Which of the following statements is (are) most accurate in defining regional cardiac dilatation after acute myocardial infarction?
    1. occurs late in the course of the post-MI period
    2. may be a lethal consequence of transmural infarcts
    3. usually occurs with inferior wall MIs
    4. it is an important mechanism of acute cardiac dilatation after myocardial infarction
    REF: N. Engl. J. Med. 300:57-62, 1979

61. Sequential radionuclide assessment of left and right ventricular performance after acute transmural myocardial infarction is likely to reveal
    1. greater reduction in right ventricular ejection fraction in inferior than anterior infarction
    2. stable ventricular systolic performance during the hospital phase of uncomplicated transmural infarction
    3. production of a greater depression in left ventricular ejection fraction with anterior than inferior infarction
    4. greater regional wall motion in anterior than inferior wall infarcts
    REF: Ann. Intern. Med. 89:441-447, 1978

62. Which of the following should be used early in the treatment of pericardial disease?
    1. symptomatic tratment in benign types of pericardial disease
    2. relief of anxiety by reassurance
    3. use of nonsteroidal anti-inflammatory drugs
    4. corticosteroids
    REF: Mod. Concepts Cardiovasc. Dis. 48:1-6, 1979

Directions Summarized				
A	B	C	D	E
1, 2, 3 only	1, 3 only	2, 4 only	4 only	All are correct

63. When using propranolol in the treatment of hypertension
    1. dosage must be individualized
    2. the starting total daily dose should not exceed 20 mg
    3. ordinarily the drug is used in conjunction with or in addition to a diuretic
    4. older patients respond better than do younger patients
    REF: Curr. Probl. Cardiol. 3 (No. 10):1-53, 1979

64. In the treatment of hypertension the advantages of β-blockers include(s)
    1. sedative effect
    2. patient acceptance
    3. postural hypotension
    4. twice daily administration
    REF: Ibid.

65. Which of the following pathogenic viruses has (have) been isolated repeatedly from human cardiac tissues?
    1. Coxsackie
    2. poliomyelitis
    3. ECHO
    4. rhinovirus
    REF: Kawai, C., Matsumori, A., Kitaura, Y. and Takatsu, T.: Viruses and the heart: viral myocarditis and cardiomyopathy. In: Yu, P.N. and Goodwin, J.F., *Progress in Cardiology, Vol. 7*, Lea & Febiger, Philadelphia, 1978, pp. 141-162

Cardiology / 17

66. Which of the following is (are) a mode(s) of presentation of viral myocarditis?
    1. pericardial rub
    2. atrial tachycardia
    3. gallop rhythms
    4. no clinical manifestations
    REF: Ibid.

67. Which of the following is (are) used in the treatment of viral myocarditis?
    1. oxygenation
    2. exercise
    3. adequate ventilation
    4. antibiotics
    REF: Ibid.

68. In a patient with angina pectoris, which of the following indications for coronary artery bypass surgery would result in a better prognosis?
    1. chronic stable angina pectoris
    2. two-vessel disease
    3. single-vessel disease
    4. main left coronary disease
    REF: Bristow, J.W.: A cardiologist's view of coronary bypass surgery. In: Yu, P.N. and Goodwin, J.F., *Progress in Cardiology, Vol. 6*, Lea & Febiger, Philadelphia, 1977, pp. 1-40

69. The features of the syndrome of sudden cardiac death include
    1. ischemic heart disease
    2. acute myocardial infarction in 20%
    3. instantaneous onset
    4. prodromes
    REF: Am. J. Cardiol. 43:313-328, 1979

	Directions Summarized			
A	B	C	D	E
1, 2, 3 only	1, 3 only	2, 4 only	4 only	All are correct

70. Which of the following is (are) a mechanism(s) of action of the vasodilator drugs in congestive heart failure?
    1. dilatation of the veins, decreasing venous return
    2. increase in the afterload of the heart
    3. increase in the stroke volume
    4. increase in the coronary driving pressure
    REF: Am. Heart J. 97:519-526, 1979

71. Which of the following vasodilator agents has (have) both arterial and venous sites of action?
    1. nitroprusside
    2. trimethaphan
    3. prazosin
    4. nitroglycerin
    REF: Ibid.

72. Which of the following is (are) clinical correlate(s) of myocardial oxygen demand?
    1. double product (heart rate × systolic blood pressure)
    2. tension-time index (heart rate × integral of left ventricular pressure during systole)
    3. triple product (heart rate × systolic blood pressure × systolic ejection time)
    4. transmural diastolic pressure gradient (aortic diastolic pressure — left ventricular diastolic pressure)
    REF: Am. Heart J. 97:527-534, 1979

Cardiology / 19

73. Which of the following parameters is increased when measured during maximal exercise in physically trained patients with coronary disease?
    1. maximum O_2 uptake
    2. work capacity
    3. maximum heart rate
    4. maximum A-V O_2 difference
    REF: Ibid.

74. Which of the following diseases can be simulated by left atrial myxomas?
    1. myocarditis
    2. mitral regurgitation
    3. infective endocarditis
    4. paroxysmal atrial tachycardia
    REF: Am. Heart J. 97:639-643, 1979

75. Which of the following factors promote(s) myocardial potassium loss and arrhythmias?
    1. ischemia and infarction
    2. catecholamine stimulation
    3. direct current countershock
    4. rapid atrial tachycardia
    REF: Am. J. Cardiol. 43:131-148, 1979

76. Which of the following antiarrhythmic factors decrease(s) myocardial potassium loss?
    1. procainamide
    2. lidocaine
    3. propranolol
    4. quinidine
    REF: Ibid.

20 / Cardiology

Directions Summarized				
A	B	C	D	E
1, 2, 3	1, 3	2, 4	4	All are
only	only	only	only	correct

77. Which of the following may result in failure of clinical response to the most appropriate antibiotics in bacterial endocarditis?
    1. delay in starting therapy
    2. suboptimal doses
    3. minimal duration of therapy
    4. local or metastatic abscesses
    REF: Am. Heart J. 96:263-269, 1978

78. Which of the following antibiotics is (are) most frequently used in *Streptococcus viridans* bacterial endocarditis?
    1. vancomycin
    2. penicillin
    3. cephalothin
    4. clindamycin
    REF: Ibid.

79. In acute myocardial infarction with left ventricular failure, nitroglycerin
    1. decreases left ventricular end-diastolic pressure
    2. decreases collateral flow
    3. decreases pulmonary capillary wedge pressure
    4. increases coronary collateral flow resistance
    REF: Am. Heart J. 96:550-553, 1978

80. In left ventricular failure, nitroglycerin
    1. reduces afterload
    2. increases left ventricular contractility
    3. decreases left ventricular end-diastolic pressure
    4. increases myocardial oxygen consumption
    REF: Ibid.

81. Spironolactone is indicated in
    1. hypercalcemia
    2. congestive heart failure
    3. renal failure
    4. hypertension
    REF: Am. Heart J. 96:824-827, 1978

82. Furosemide is most useful in
    1. hypertension
    2. cirrhosis
    3. renal failure
    4. congestive heart failure
    REF: Ibid.

83. Thiazides are most effective in treating
    1. hypertension
    2. renal failure
    3. hypercalcemia
    4. congestive heart failure
    REF: Ibid.

84. Which of the following is (are) an ECG criterion (criteria) for an abnormal exercise electrocardiogram?
    1. 1.0 mm horizontal or down-sloping ST depression
    2. T-wave inversion
    3. ST-segment elevation
    4. 0.08 second duration ST-segment depression
    REF: Am. Heart J. 95:102-114, 1978

85. Prazosin produces a(n)
    1. reflex tachycardia
    2. decrease in blood pressure
    3. increase in renin release
    4. sympathetic blockade
    REF: Am. Heart J. 95:262-265, 1978

Directions Summarized				
A	B	C	D	E
1, 2, 3 only	1, 3 only	2, 4 only	4 only	All are correct

86. Which of the following drugs is (are) used for hypertensive emergencies?
    1. diazoxide
    2. prazosin
    3. sodium nitroprusside
    4. thiazides
    REF: Am. Heart J. 95:389-393, 1978

87. Although effective, cheap, and available in many forms, thiazide diuretics
    1. accentuate diabetes
    2. produce gout
    3. cause gastrointestinal disturbances
    4. produce potassium loss
    REF: Ibid.

88. Which of the following groups of drugs may be hazardous in the treatment of shock in acute myocardial infarction?
    1. vasodilators
    2. diuretics
    3. inotropic agents
    4. vasopressors
    REF: Am. Heart J. 95:529-534, 1978

89. In the treatment of angina pectoris propranolol and nitrates combined produce the following hemodynamic and other alterations
    1. increased heart rate
    2. increased cardiac output
    3. increased systemic arterial pressure
    4. increased left ventricular volume
    REF: Am. Heart J. 95:775-788, 1978

90. Smoking cigarettes can serve as a precipitating factor in angina pectoris due to the following physiologic factors
    1. increased blood oxygen content
    2. increased heart rate
    3. decreased diastolic arterial pressure
    4. depressed left ventricular function
    REF: Ibid.

91. Physical conditioning in the patient with angina pectoris
    1. enhances left ventricular performance
    2. produces greater oxygen extraction by skeletal muscle
    3. reduces plasma catecholamine levels during exercise
    4. enhances direct cardiac effects
    REF: Ibid.

92. Which of the following is (are) an effect(s) of severe magnesium deficiency on the ECG?
    1. prolonged PR interval
    2. widened QRS
    3. depressed ST segment
    4. peaked T wave
    REF: Am. Heart J. 94:649-657, 1977

93. Which of the following statements concerning bacterial shock is (are) correct?
    1. the majority of cases is caused by gram-negative enteric bacilli
    2. diabetes, chronic liver disease, and blood dyscrasias predispose to bacteremia and shock
    3. bacteremia with shock is usually precipitated by a manipulative procedure
    4. treatment with corticosteroids, immunosuppressive drugs, and antimetabolites predispose to sepsis
    REF: Am. Heart J. 94:112-114, 1977

Directions Summarized				
A	B	C	D	E
1, 2, 3 only	1, 3 only	2, 4 only	4 only	All are correct

94. Which of the following disease entities demonstrate(s) abnormal ventricular septal motion on M-mode echocardiography?
    1. pulmonic stenosis
    2. coronary artery disease
    3. tricuspid valve replacement
    4. severe left ventricular dysfunction
    REF: Am. Heart J. 94:227-249, 1977

95. In a patient with pacemaker malfunction, the chest x-ray can demonstrate
    1. unequivocal displacement of the lead within the heart
    2. lifting of infected myocardial electrodes from the surface of the heart
    3. fractured intramyocardial lead
    4. Twidlers syndrome
    REF: Am. Heart J. 94:378-386, 1977

96. Which of the following factors is (are) responsible for malfunction of the lead system in cardiac pacemakers?
    1. insulation
    2. poor sensing
    3. high threshold
    4. poor position
    REF: Ibid.

97. Intimal fibrous proliferation in saphenous veins used for aortocoronary bypass grafts can be caused by
    1. medial ischemia
    2. thrombosis
    3. adventitial ischemia
    4. increased wall O_2 tension
    REF: Am. Heart J. 94:500-516, 1977

98. The optimal management of hypertrophic obstructive cardiomyopathy is
    1. myectomy
    2. complete β-blockade
    3. ventriculomyotomy
    4. control of arrhythmias
    REF: Am. J. Cardiol. 42:993-1001, 1978

99. The ability to terminate reentry tachycardias with timed stimuli is affected by which of the following factors?
    1. the size and site of the tachycardia circuit
    2. the distance between the site of stimulation and the site of the tachycardia circuit
    3. the heart rate during tachycardia
    4. the electrophysiologic properties of the tissues between the site of stimulation and the tachycardia circuit
    REF: Am. J. Cardiol. 41:1025-1034, 1978

100. Which of the following ECG findings can be present in patients with vasospastic acute myocardial ischemia?
    1. ST-segment elevation
    2. ST-segment depression
    3. pseudonormalization of T waves
    4. decrease in T-wave voltage
    REF: Am. J. Cardiol. 42:1019-1035, 1978

II: Hematology

DIRECTIONS: Each of the questions or incomplete statements below is followed by four or five suggested answers or completions. Select the **one** that is **BEST** in each case.

1. The most benign type of non-Hodgkin's lymphomas is
   A. nodular lymphoma
   B. diffuse lymphocytic lymphoma
   C. diffuse mixed histiocytic-lymphocytic lymphoma
   D. histiocytic lymphoma
   REF: Erslev, A.J. and Gabuzda, T.G.: *Pathophysiology of Blood, 2nd Ed.,* W.B. Saunders Company, Philadelphia, 1979, p. 152
   Cancer 39:999, 1977

2. The most benign type of Hodgkin's lymphoma is
   A. lymphocyte depletion
   B. mixed cellularity
   C. nodular sclerosis
   D. lymphocyte predominance
   REF: Erslev, A.J. and Gabuzda, T.G.: *Pathophysiology of Blood, 2nd Ed.,* W.B. Saunders Company, Philadelphia, 1979, p. 151

3. A favorable prognosis in Hodgkin's lymphoma is determined by
   A. the presence or absence of Reed-Sternberg cells
   B. age
   C. sex
   D. preservation or depletion of lymphocytes
   REF: Ibid., p. 150

4. The heterophil antibody typically found in patients with infectious mononucleosis is a plasma IgM macroglobulin that agglutinates sheep erythrocytes and may be removed from plasma or serum by
   A. absorption with beef erythrocytes but not with guinea pig kidney cells
   B. absorption with both beef erythrocytes and guinea pig kidney cells
   C. absorption with guinea pig kidney cells but not with beef erythrocytes
   D. absorption with neither beef erythrocytes nor guinea pig kidney cells
   REF: Lichtman, M.A. (Ed.): *Hematology for Practitioners,* Little, Brown and Company, Boston, 1978, p. 182

5. Unfavorable prognostic signs during the course of chronic myelogenous leukemia include
   A. enlarged superficial lymph nodes
   B. fever
   C. destructive bone lesions
   D. pronounced basophilia or eosinophilia
   E. all of the above
   REF: Williams, W.J., Beutler, E., Erslev, A.J. and Rundles, R.W. (Eds.): *Hematology, 2nd Ed.,* McGraw-Hill Book Company, New York, 1977, p. 789

6. In which of the following does the abnormal cell contain thromboplastic substances that can be released into the bloodstream and can activate the soluble coagulation factors?
   A. acute myelocytic leukemia
   B. erythroleukemia
   C. acute promyelocytic leukemia
   D. acute lymphocytic leukemia
   E. preleukemia
   REF: Reich, P.R.: *Hematology: Physiopathologic Basis for Clinical Practice,* Little, Brown and Company, Boston, 1978, p. 285

7. The lymphocytes in acute lymphocytic leukemia usually lack
   A. B-lymphocyte markers
   B. T-lymphocyte markers
   C. both B- and T-cell markers
   D. neither B- nor T-cell markers
   REF: Ibid., p. 294

8. Immunologic and biochemical assays for TdT (terminal deoxynucleotidyl transferase) are useful in
   A. confirming the diagnosis of acute lymphoblastic leukemia
   B. evaluating patients with blastic transformation of chronic granulocytic leukemia
   C. distinguishing lymphoblastic lymphoma from other poorly differentiated lymphomas
   D. all of the above
   E. only A and C
   REF: Erslev, A.J. and Gabuzda, T.G.: *Pathophysiology of Blood, 2nd Ed.,* W.B. Saunders Company, Philadelphia, 1979, p. 147

9. In what percent of patients with multiple myeloma does amyloidosis occur?
   A. 2%
   B. 7%
   C. 20%
   D. 35%
   REF: Lichtman, M.A. (Ed.): *Hematology for Practitioners,* Little, Brown and Company, Boston, 1978, p. 265

10. Chemotherapeutic agents of greatest value in the treatment of Hodgkin's disease include
   A. alkylating agents
   B. vinca alkaloids
   C. procarbazine
   D. adrenal glucocorticoids
   E. all of the above
   REF: Erslev, A.J. and Gabuzda, T.G.: *Pathophysiology of Blood, 2nd Ed.,* W.B. Saunders Company, Philadelphia, 1979, p. 150

11. Aspirin inhibits platelet aggregation by
   A. inhibiting phospholipase A_2 needed in synthesizing arachidonic acid from membrane phospholipids
   B. inhibiting cyclooxygenase, which transforms arachidonic acid to cyclic endoperoxides
   C. inhibiting thromboxane synthetase required for the synthesis of thromboxanes from endoperoxides
   D. inhibiting a synthetase needed for the synthesis of prostacyclin from cyclic endoperoxides
   REF: Ibid., p. 159
   N. Engl. J. Med. 297:1386, 1977

12. Nonimmune peripheral destruction of platelets occurs in
   A. neonatal thrombocytopenia
   B. idiopathic thrombocytopenic purpura
   C. thrombotic thrombocytopenic purpura
   D. quinidine-induced thrombocytopenia
   E. thrombocytopenia secondary to SLE
   REF: Lichtman, M.A. (Ed.): *Hematology for Practitioners,* Little, Brown and Company, Boston, 1978, p. 286

13. Von Willebrand's disease is an inherited disorder of primary hemostasis characterized by
    A. diminished levels of Factor VIII protein
    B. decreased coagulant properties of Factor VIII
    C. decreased platelet adherence promoting activity of Factor VIII
    D. all of the above
    E. only B and C
    REF: Reich, P.R.: *Hematology: Physiopathologic Basis for Clinical Practice,* Little, Brown and Company, Boston, 1978, p. 403

14. Idiopathic thrombocythemia (autonomous thrombocytosis) is a primary marrow disorder characterized by
    A. small megakaryocytes with diminished cytoplasmic mass and ploidy
    B. lack of bleeding or thrombotic episodes
    C. abnormal platelets that do not aggregate normally in response to epinephrine and ADP
    D. occurrence in nonhematologic malignancies
    REF: Ibid., pp. 402-403

15. Hemarthroses are the most frequent indication for admitting patients with hemophilia A to the hospital. The joint that is most frequently involved in hemarthroses is the
    A. wrist
    B. elbow
    C. hip
    D. knee
    E. ankle
    REF: Williams, W.J., Beutler, E., Erslev, A.J., and Rundles, R.W. (Eds.): *Hematology, 2nd Ed.,* McGraw-Hill Book Company, New York, 1977, p. 1408

32 / Hematology

16. One of the major causes of death in hemophilia A is
A. hemorrhage into the gastrointestinal tract
B. hemorrhage into the upper respiratory tract
C. hemorrhage within the intracranial cavity
D. hemorrhage into the retroperitoneum
E. the development of circulating anti-Factor VIII antibody
REF: Ibid.

17. The most recent and most promising mode of therapy for thrombotic thrombocytopenic purpura (TTP) and the hemolytic uremia syndrome is
A. the use of glucocorticoids followed by splenectomy
B. the use of low-dose heparin followed by splenectomy
C. the use of antiplatelet drugs such as aspirin and persantin
D. exchange transfusions and plasma infusions
REF: Erslev, A.J. and Gabuzda, T.G.: *Pathophysiology of Blood, 2nd Ed.,* W.B. Saunders Company, Philadelphia, 1979, p. 169

18. Heparin is rapidly cleared from the circulation with a half-life of
A. 45 minutes
B. 90 minutes
C. 150 minutes
D. 3 hours
E. 4 hours
REF: Ibid., p. 179

19. Disseminated intravascular coagulation is a bleeding disorder in which some or all of the following may be present EXCEPT
A. hyperfibrinogenemia
B. thrombocytopenia
C. red-cell fragmentation
D. increased levels of fibrin split products
E. reduced Factor V and VIII levels
REF: Lichtman, M.A. (Ed.): *Hematology for Practitioners,* Little, Brown and Company, Boston, 1978, p. 311

20. The most common cause of excessive bleeding after cardiopulmonary bypass surgery is
    A. defective sutures at the site of surgery
    B. excess heparin
    C. dilutional coagulopathy due to massive transfusion with three-day-old blood
    D. acute DIC
    E. none of the above
    REF: Ibid., pp. 317-318

21. All of the following are important causes of iron deficiency in adults EXCEPT
    A. subtotal gastrectomy
    B. pregnancy
    C. poor dietary intake of iron
    D. hereditary hemorrhagic telangiectasia
    E. hookworm infestation
    REF: Reich, P.R.: *Hematology: Physiopathologic Basis for Clinical Practice,* Little, Brown and Company, Boston, 1978, pp. 40-42

22. The most common cause of a positive indirect Coombs' test and a concomitantly negative direct Coombs' test is
    A. idiopathic autoimmune hemolytic anemia
    B. drug-induced hemolytic anemia
    C. alloimmunization secondary to previous exposure to "nonself" erythrocytic antigens
    D. secondary autoimmune hemolytic anemia
    E. none of the above
    REF: Ibid., p. 128

34 / Hematology

23. Hereditary spherocytosis (HS) is characterized by all of the following EXCEPT
    A. polychromatophilia and reticulocytosis in peripheral blood
    B. erythroid hyperplasia of the bone marrow
    C. splenomegaly
    D. increased osmotic resistance of erythrocytes
    E. autosomal dominant inheritance
    REF: Erslev, A.J. and Gabuzda, T.G.: *Pathophysiology of Blood, 2nd Ed.,* W.B. Saunders Company, Philadelphia, 1979, p. 95

24. Which of the following items is of least value in the differential diagnosis of polycythemia vera from polycythemia secondary to chronic pulmonary disease?
    A. determination of arterial blood gases
    B. history and physical examination
    C. determination of serum or urine erythropoietin level
    D. determination of blood volume
    E. determination of leukocyte alkaline phosphatase score
    REF: Ibid., p. 40

25. A young man with sickle cell trait (AS) marries a woman with hemoglobin SC disease. Which of the following is most likely for children of this marriage?
    A. all children will have sickle cell trait (AS)
    B. there is a 25% probability that the child will have a normal hemoglobin pattern (AA)
    C. all children will have sickle cell anemia (SS)
    D. all children will have Hb C trait (AC)
    E. there is a 25% probability that children will have sickle cell anemia
    REF: Williams, W.J., Beutler, E., Erslev, A.J. and Rundles, R.W. (Eds.): *Hematology, 2nd Ed.,* McGraw-Hill Book Company, New York, 1977, p. 495

26. In thymoma, what percent of cases is associated with pure red-cell aplasia?
   A. 5%
   B. 15%
   C. 35%
   D. 50%
   E. 75%
   REF: Lichtman, M.A. (Ed.): *Hematology for Practitioners,* Little, Brown and Company, Boston, 1978, p. 42

27. Pernicious anemia is the disease most often associated with vitamin B_{12} deficiency. The basic defect in this disease is
   A. inability to secrete hydrochloric acid even after parenteral stimulation with histamine or betazole
   B. congenital intrinsic factor deficiency
   C. defective secretion of intrinsic factor by the gastric mucosal cell owing to the presence of blocking or precipitating antibodies
   D. selective malabsorption of vitamin B_{12} due to congenital absence of the ileal receptor for the intrinsic factor-B_{12} complex
   REF: Reich, P.R.: *Hematology: Physiopathologic Basis for Clinical Practice,* Little, Brown and Company, Boston, 1978, p. 74

28. Modes of therapy in homozygous β-thalassemia (Cooley's anemia) include
   A. blood transfusion
   B. splenectomy
   C. folic acid
   D. parenteral administration of iron-chelating agents such as desferrioxamine
   E. all of the above
   REF: Ibid., p. 179

36 / Hematology

29. All of the following items concerning pyruvate kinase deficiency are true EXCEPT
- A. irregularly contracted cells or burr cells may be prominent
- B. spherocytes are rare or absent
- C. the unincubated osmotic fragility is abnormal
- D. aplastic crises can occur in association with infection
- E. splenomegaly may be present

REF: Ibid., p. 159

30. The anemia most commonly present in systemic lupus erythematosus is
- A. autoimmune hemolytic anemia
- B. normochromic and normocytic anemia of chronic disease
- C. iron-deficiency anemia
- D. microangiopathic hemolytic anemia
- E. pure red-cell aplasia

REF: Ibid., p. 238

DIRECTIONS: For each of the following questions or incomplete statements, **ONE** or **MORE** of the answers or completions given is correct. Select:
- A if only 1, 2 and 3 are correct,
- B if only 1 and 3 are correct,
- C if only 2 and 4 are correct,
- D if only 4 is correct,
- E if all are correct.

---

31. Cold agglutinating antibodies against I antigen may appear following
1. influenza pneumonia
2. infectious mononucleosis
3. *Mycoplasma pneumoniae*
4. *Escherichia coli* septicemia

REF: Ibid., p. 222

32. Noninvasive and portable procedures that are well suited for diagnosing large-vessel (popliteal and femoral) disease but are less reliable for calf vein thrombosis include
    1. ^{125}I-fibrinogen uptake
    2. Doppler ultrasonography
    3. venography
    4. impedance plethysmography
    REF: Lichtman, M.A. (Ed.): *Hematology for Practitioners,* Little, Brown and Company, Boston, 1978, p. 327

33. Reticulocytosis occurs in the following types of anemia
    1. fragmentation hemolysis
    2. hereditary spherocytosis
    3. immune hemolytic disease
    4. sickle cell anemia during an aplastic crisis due to viral infection
    REF: Ibid., pp. 51-58

34. Extraction of one or two teeth in a patient with hemophilia A should be accompanied by
    1. raising Factor VIII level to 50%
    2. application of a protective acrylic splint
    3. administration of epsilon-aminocaproic acid 24 gm per day *po* for 10 days
    4. antibiotic therapy
    REF: Williams, W.J., Beutler, E., Erslev, A.J. and Rundles, R.W. (Eds.): *Hematology, 2nd Ed.,* McGraw-Hill Book Company, New York, 1977, p. 1413

35. Microangiopathic hemolytic anemia may be secondary to
    1. thrombotic thrombocytopenic purpura
    2. renal transplantation rejection
    3. disseminated intravascular coagulation
    4. scleroderma
    REF: Lichtman, M.A. (Ed.): *Hematology for Practitioners,* Little, Brown and Company, Boston, 1978, p. 68

Directions Summarized				
A	B	C	D	E
1, 2, 3 only	1, 3 only	2, 4 only	4 only	All are correct

36. Bence Jones protein is best described as
    1. a cryoglobulin
    2. a pyroglobulin
    3. an agglutinin
    4. an L (light) chain
    REF: Reich, P.R.: *Hematology: Physiopathologic Basis for Clinical Practice,* Little, Brown and Company, Boston, 1978, p. 376

37. In acute myelocytic leukemia, induction is usually attempted with
    1. vincristine
    2. daunomycin
    3. melphalan
    4. cytosine arabinoside
    REF: Ibid., p. 299

38. Drugs that may potentiate the effects of coumarin include
    1. salicylates
    2. allopurinol
    3. quinidine
    4. rifampin
    REF: Williams, W.J., Beutler, E., Erslev, A.J. and Rundles, R.W. (Eds.): *Hematology, 2nd Ed.,* McGraw-Hill Book Company, New York, 1977, p. 1485

39. T-cell neoplasias include
1. chronic lymphocytic leukemia
2. mycosis fungoides
3. most of the non-Hodgkin's lymphomas
4. Sézary syndrome
REF: Erslev, A.J. and Gabuzda, T.G.: *Pathophysiology of Blood, 2nd Ed.*, W.B. Saunders Company, Philadelphia, 1979, p. 145

40. Therapy for aplastic anemia may include
1. blood transfusion
2. androgens
3. glucocorticoids
4. bone marrow transplantation
REF: Lichtman, M.A. (Ed.): *Hematology for Practitioners*, Little, Brown and Company, Boston, 1978, p. 126

III: Neurology

DIRECTIONS: Each of the questions or incomplete statements below is followed by five suggested answers or completions. Select the **one** that is **BEST** in each case.

1. The most common neurologic involvement in Paget's disease is
   A. cranial nerve VII
   B. cranial nerve VIII
   C. the spinal cord
   D. the spinal roots and nerves
   E. none of the above
   REF: Neurology 29:448, 1979

2. The most common area of headache in children with migraine is
   A. bilateral frontal
   B. unilateral frontal
   C. posterior
   D. bilateral temporal
   E. unilateral temporal
   REF: Ibid., p. 507

3. All are true regarding cerebral infarction in young adults, EXCEPT
   A. two thirds of patients will recover or improve to functional independence
   B. premature atherosclerotic disease and hypertension play a role
   C. cerebral embolism of cardiac origin is a frequent cause
   D. the etiology can be identified in over half of the cases
   E. occlusive extracranial vascular disease is the leading cause
   REF: Stroke 9:39, 1978

4. The consistent features of capsular infarcts include
   A. a purely motor hemiparesis
   B. hemiparesis plus sensory loss
   C. hemiparesis plus homonymous hemianopsia
   D. hemiparesis with prolonged aphasia (in dominant hemisphere)
   E. C and D only
   REF: Arch. Neurol. 36:73, 1979

5. Focal motor and generalized epilepsy treatment with carbamazepine or phenytoin show
   A. better seizure control with carbamazepine
   B. more acute side effects with carbamazepine
   C. better seizure control with phenytoin
   D. more acute side effects with phenytoin
   E. none of the above
   REF: Ibid., p. 22

6. Early Huntington's disease is characterized by all of the following EXCEPT
   A. low IQ
   B. impaired memory quotients
   C. impaired short-term memory
   D. impaired retrieval from long-term memory
   E. choreiform movements
   REF: Arch. Neurol. 35:585, 1978

7. Severe dementia occurs in approximately what percent of the population over age 65?
   A. 1%
   B. 4–5%
   C. 11–12%
   D. 17%
   E. 31%
   REF: Tyler, H.R. and Dawson, D.M. (Eds.): *Current Neurology, Vol. 1,* Houghton Mifflin, Boston, 1978, p. 361

8. The prevalence of Parkinson's disease in the United States is approximately
   A. 0.5/1,000
   B. 2/1,000
   C. 3.5/1,000
   D. 5/1,000
   E. none of the above
   REF: Ibid., p. 363

9. The most common clinical findings in patients with Alzheimer's disease, in decreasing order of frequency, are
   A. memory loss, disorientation, agitation
   B. agitation, dysphasia, disorientation
   C. memory loss, dyspraxia, gait disturbance
   D. agitation, memory loss, dyspraxia
   E. incontinence, disorientation, memory loss
   REF: Ibid., p. 365

10. Neurologic complications of cardiac catheterization commonly are of which type and occur in which location?
    A. thrombotic, in the right hemisphere
    B. hemorrhagic, in the basal ganglia
    C. embolic, in the brainstem
    D. thrombotic, in the brainstem
    E. hemorrhagic, in the left hemisphere
    REF: Ibid., p. 469

11. With mitral valve prolapse
    A. small strokes occur in nearly one third of patients
    B. strokes, when they occur, are usually embolic
    C. auricular fibrillation increases the risk of embolism
    D. B and C occur
    E. A, B, and C occur
    REF: Ibid., p. 469

12. Features of adrenoleukodystrophy include
    A. pronounced skin pallor
    B. reduced adrenal reserve
    C. probable abnormal fatty acid synthesis
    D. A and B
    E. A, B, and C
    REF: Ibid, p. 471

13. Which of the following statements is (are) applicable to strionigral degeneration?
    A. does not respond as well to levodopa as does paralysis agitans
    B. usually presents with an asymmetrical parkinsonian syndrome
    C. may mimic Shy-Drager syndrome
    D. A and C
    E. A, B, and C
    REF: Ibid., p. 113

14. Shy-Drager syndrome and parkinsonism have certain features in common. Which of the following is NOT true?
    A. both may have bradykinesias
    B. both show hypersensitivity to intravenous norepinephrine
    C. both show hypersensitivity to intravenous dopamine
    D. Shy-Drager patients may show more improvement than Parkinson patients on fluorocortisone therapy
    E. levodopa is more effective for parkinsonism than for Shy-Drager syndrome
    REF: Ibid., p. 114

15. Which of the following statements apply to hypertension headache?
    A. may occur with acute as well as chronic hypertension
    B. represents a very small percentage of headaches in the general population
    C. has a well-understood pathogenesis
    D. A and B
    E. A and C
    REF: Ibid., pp. 197-198

16. All are true of hypertensive encephalopathy EXCEPT
    A. it appears to be decreasing in incidence
    B. it has been affecting a smaller number of older patients in recent years
    C. hypertension of any origin may produce it
    D. papilledema is generally proportional to the increase in intracranial pressure
    E. convulsions are common with this condition
    REF: Ibid., p. 199

17. Intracranial aneurysms have the folowing characteristics, EXCEPT
    A. there is a gradual increase in the overall prevalence
    B. they are slightly more common in females
    C. the highest likelihood of rupture is in the sixth decade
    D. about 2% occur in children or adolescents
    E. surgical treatment has been found superior to conservative management in alert patients, whether adults or children
    REF: Ibid., pp. 223, 236

18. The neurologic complications of 5-fluorouracil therapy
    A. occur in 15%-20% of patients with "conventional" doses of 15 mg/kg
    B. affect mainly the basal ganglia and peripheral nerves
    C. are related to the total dose rather than the dose given at each administration
    D. none of the above
    E. A, B, and C
    REF: Ibid., p. 313

DIRECTIONS: For each of the following questions or incomplete statements, **ONE** or **MORE** of the answers or completions given is correct. Select:
- **A** if only 1, 2 and 3 are correct,
- **B** if only 1 and 3 are correct,
- **C** if only 2 and 4 are correct,
- **D** if only 4 is correct,
- **E** if all are correct

19. Partial seizures with complex symptomatology
    1. are also known as psychomotor seizures
    2. respond best to ethosuximide
    3. respond about equally to carbamazepine and phenytoin
    4. should never be treated with temporal lobectomy
    REF: Ibid., p. 247

20. Regarding anticonvulsants
    1. trimethadione is effective for grand mal attacks
    2. valproate is effective for petit mal and some grand mal seizures
    3. phenytoin is rapidly effective if given intramuscularly
    4. primidone is partially metabolized to phenobarbital
    REF: Ibid., pp. 247–252

21. In response to a standardized exercise test
    1. the correlation of changes in blood lactate, creatinine kinase, and fatty acids may be of diagnostic value
    2. patients with a disproportionate rise in creatinine kinase may have metabolic myopathies
    3. patients with a disproportionate rise of lactate may have mitochondrial abnormalities
    4. normals do not show a rise of lactate or creatinine kinase
    REF: Neurology 29:636, 1979

22. Facial myokymia
    1. is an intermittent twitching of muscles of the face
    2. is less common than myokymia of the upper extermity
    3. is most often seen with polyradiculoneuropathy
    4. is associated with multiple sclerosis or brainstem neoplasms
    REF: Ibid., p. 662

23. Unilateral neglect (hemi-inattention) may result from lesions in the
    1. parietal lobe
    2. putamen
    3. gyrus cinguli
    4. thalamus
    REF: Ibid., p. 690

24. Vincristine
    1. almost always causes a peripheral neuropathy
    2. spares the autonomic nervous system as a rule
    3. therapy may be accompanied by seizures, but the causal relationship is unclear
    4. has an effective antidote to minimize its toxicity
    REF: Tyler, H.R. and Dawson, D.M. (Eds.): *Current Neurology, Vol. 1*, Houghton Mifflin, Boston, 1978, pp. 307–311

25. Effects of phenytoin on bone and vitamin D metabolism include
    1. a decrease in serum calcium
    2. a decrease in serum albumin
    3. a decrease in serum 25-hydroxycholecalciferol
    4. an increase in serum alkaline phosphatase
    REF: Ann. Neurol. 5:374, 1979

Directions Summarized				
A	B	C	D	E
1, 2, 3 only	1, 3 only	2, 4 only	4 only	All are correct

26. In a series of computed tomography scans of the brain in patients with CNS lupus, the findings demonstrate
    1. sulcal enlargement is most common
    2. subdural hematomas are nearly as common as infarcts
    3. ventricular enlargement is common
    4. infarcts and intracerebral hemorrhages are rare
    REF: Ibid., p. 158

27. Regarding human brain weights
    1. male and female brain weights are nearly equal
    2. the largest increase in brain weight occurs during the first three years of life
    3. brain weight begins to decline at 25 years of age
    4. brain weight is some 10% lower during the ninth decade than during early adult life
    REF: Ann. Neurol. 4:345, 1978

28. Regarding risk factors for cerebral complications of angiography for transient ischemic attacks and stroke
    1. patients in whom the study is most needed tend to be those at greatest risk
    2. risk is unrelated to the number of selective injections
    3. risk is strongly related to the number of previous transient ischemic attacks
    4. the degree of arterial stenosis does not affect the risk
    REF: Neurology 29:4, 1979

29. Calcification of the basal ganglia found on computerized tomography
  1. is usually asymmetric
  2. involves mainly the putamen
  3. rarely involves the globus pallidus
  4. has little pathophysiologic significance for altered calcium metabolism
  REF: Ibid., p. 328

30. Primary intracerebral hemorrhage
  1. has an incidence of about 2/100,000 population per year
  2. is more common in females than in males
  3. decreases after age 50
  4. has decreased gradually in incidence during the past 30 years
  REF: Ann. Neurol. 5:367, 1979

IV: Infectious Diseases

DIRECTIONS: Each of the questions or incomplete statements below is followed by five suggested answers of completions. Select the **one** that is **BEST** in each case.

1. Bacterial etiology of intra-abdominal abscesses most commonly includes all of the following organisms EXCEPT
   A. *Escherichia coli*
   B. *Clostridium perfringens*
   C. anaerobic streptococci
   D. *Bacteroides* sps.
   E. *Klebsiella-Aerobacter* group
   REF: Am. J. Surg. 125:70–78, 1973

2. Which of the following statements about tetanus is INCORRECT?
   A. *Clostridium tetani* is a gram-positive, anaerobic, slender motile rod
   B. sporulation takes place only *in vitro* and not in tissues
   C. spores may survive in soil for years
   D. all of the clinical features are produced by a neurotoxin tetanospasmin
   E. only vegetable forms and not spores produce toxin
   REF: N. Engl. J. Med. 289:1293–1296, 1973

3. Which of the following organisms is the most frequently isolated etiologic agent from heroin addicts with endocarditis?
   A. *Staphylococcus aureus*
   B. *Staphylococcus epidermidis*
   C. Pseudomonas species
   D. Candida species
   E. Streptococcus species
   REF: Ann. Intern. Med. 18:699-702, 1973

4. Which of the following parasites does NOT seem to produce an increased incidence of infection in steroid-treated patients?
   A. *Toxoplasma gondii*
   B. *Ascaris lumbricoides*
   C. *Pneumocystis carinii*
   D. Malaria
   E. *Entamoeba histolytica*
   REF: Med. Clin. North Am. 57:1277–1287, 1973

52 / Infectious Diseases

5. Each of the following statements about infection in patients with multiple myeloma is true EXCEPT
   A. there appears to be an increased frequency of gram-negative infections in patients with multiple myeloma
   B. corticosteroid therapy increases the risk of infection
   C. serum IgG levels are invariably depressed in infected myeloma patients
   D. antibody reponses to antigenic stimulation are poor in these patients
   E. complement activity is usually normal
   REF: Am. J. Med. 52:87-92, 1972

6. The role of underlying illnesses in the outcome of gram-negative infections can be summarized by all of the following EXCEPT
   A. relatively few patients with potentially curable lesions develop sepsis
   B. in acute leukemia, gram-positive infection is more lethal than gram-negative infection
   C. upper and lower respiratory tract neoplasms predispose the patient to gram-negative pneumonitides
   D. granulocytopenic patients die more frequently from an infection with gram-negative than gram-positive organisms
   E. a high mortality in gram-negative infections is associated with intravascular coagulation, uremia, and leukopenia
   REF: Eur. J. Cancer 9:69-76, 1973

7. Staphylococcal endocarditis may be difficult to diagnose in the geriatric patient because of all of the following EXCEPT
   A. initial symptoms are usually nonspecific, e.g., mental confusion, anorexia, weakness
   B. there is usually no history of fever
   C. cardiac murmurs may be absent and there may be no history of underlying heart disease
   D. Osler's nodes and Janeway lesions, although common, are frequently overlooked
   E. the source of staphylococcal bacteremia is usually not apparent
   REF: Geriatrics 28:168-173, 1973

8. A 36-year-old man diagnosed as having leptospirosis was started on high doses of intravenous ampicillin, following which his temperature rose abruptly from 99°F to 103 and pulse to 120/min. Following this, he remained afebrile. The most probable explanation for this is
   A. drug fever
   B. Jarisch-Herxheimer reaction
   C. incorrect diagnosis
   D. resistant organism
   E. temperature recorded incorrectly
   REF: Br. Med. J. 1:231-233, 1969

9. Each of the following manifestations correctly describe tuberculosis EXCEPT
   A. primary tuberculosis is not expressed symptomatically until lesions are quite extensive
   B. late exacerbating tuberculosis is not expressed symptomatically until lesions are quite extensive
   C. symptoms only become specific for tuberculosis late in the course of the disease
   D. most common symptoms are malaise, fatigue, anorexia, weight loss, and fever
   E. temperature is usually maximal in evening and is accompanied by night sweats
   REF: Harris, H.W. and McClement, J.H. In: Hoeprich, P.D., (Ed.), *Infectious Diseases, 2nd Ed.*, Harper & Row, Hagerstown, Md., 1977, pp. 318-342

10. The most common symptoms of brucellosis in the United States include all of the following EXCEPT
    A. intermittent fever
    B. chills
    C. orchitis
    D. diffuse myalgias
    E. sweating and weakness
    REF: Center for Disease Control: *Brucellosis Surveillance, Annual Summary 1972*, issued February, 1974

11. Which of the following statements concerning infection in patients with indwelling uterine devices (IUD) is INCORRECT?
   A. the majority of the pelvic infections are due to *Neisseria gonorrheae*
   B. duration of exposure to IUD is an important factor in development of infection
   C. there is a high incidence of anaerobic isolates
   D. foul-smelling mucoid discharge on the IUD tail may be the first clue to infection
   E. an infection with an IUD requires removal followed by antibacterial therapy
   REF: Int. J. Fertil. 18:156–160, 1973

12. Situations in which steroids may be therapeutically effective adjunctive therapy include all of the following EXCEPT
   A. typhoid fever
   B. brucellosis
   C. allergic aspergillus pneumonitis
   D. streptococcal sepsis
   E. miliary tuberculosis
   REF: Med. Clin. North Am. 57:1277–1287, 1973

13. Illnesses sometimes mistaken for botulism can be differentiated by all of the following EXCEPT
   A. common bacterial food poisoning shows diarrhea in the absence of cranial nerve involvement
   B. mushroom poisoning (*Amanita phalloides*) produces only pyramidal tract signs
   C. atropine poisoning has rapid onset, with facial flushing and bizarre hallucinations
   D. fever usually distinguishes poliomyelitis, meningitis, and encephalitis
   E. Guillain-Barré syndrome is characterized by ascending paralysis followed by cranial nerve involvement
   REF: Am. J. Clin. Pathol. 24:580–587, 1954

14. Gastrointestinal tuberculosis may be described by all of the following EXCEPT
    A. anemia, an elevated erythrocyte sedimentation rate, and leukocytosis occur frequently
    B. there are no diagnostic radiologic patterns
    C. skin test with PPD may be negative
    D. may resemble a wide variety of other clinical conditions
    E. chest x-ray shows evidence of tuberculosis in most cases
    REF: S. Afr. Med. J. 47:365-372, 1973

15. All of the following measures are of therapeutic value in clinical tetanus EXCEPT
    A. early administration of specific antitoxin
    B. surgical excision of the site at which organisms are producing toxin
    C. penicillin or another appropriate antibiotic
    D. large doses of corticosteroids
    E. barbiturates and/or phenothiazines
    REF: N. Engl. J. Med. 289:1293-1296, 1973

16. All of the following are true of Rocky Mountain spotted fever EXCEPT
    A. it is primarily a disease of childhood
    B. *Proteus* OX-K agglutinins rising greater than four-fold are diagnostic
    C. disseminated intravascular coagulation occurs frequently and carries a poor prognosis when severe
    D. neurologic abnormalities occur in over 50% of cases
    E. chloramphenicol and tetracycline are both effective therapeutically
    REF: Arch. Intern. Med. 132:340-347, 1973

17. Fever of unknown origin can be caused by an adult form of juvenile rheumatoid arthritis characterized by all of the following EXCEPT
    A. all patients are serologically positive for rheumatoid factor and antinuclear antibody
    B. lab findings usually include normochromic normocytic anemia and leukocytosis
    C. few patients have x-ray evidence of arthritis
    D. daily temperature is frequently up to or greater than 105F
    E. rash, lymphadenopathy, splenomegaly, pneumonitis, arthritis, pericarditis, and abdominal pain are characteristic
    REF: Medicine 52:431–444, 1973

18. Acute urethritis in male college students can be characterized by all of the following EXCEPT
    A. nongonococcal urethritis appears to be much more common than gonococcal urethritis in this population
    B. T-strain mycoplasmas appear to be the cause of nongonococcal urethritis
    C. symptoms of nongonococcal urethritis clear with tetracycline or erythromycin therapy
    D. post-therapy cultures of nongonococcal urethritis show a carrier rate of T-mycoplasmas equal to controls
    E. gonococci are resistant to tetracycline in this population
    REF: J.A.M.A. 226:37–39, 1973

19. All of the following correctly describe *Klebsiella pneumoniae* EXCEPT
    A. it is often associated with pneumococcal infection
    B. upper lobes are more generally involved
    C. mortality is high, occurring late in the disease
    D. alcoholism and debilitation are frequent predisposing factors
    E. bulging fissures and abscess formation are frequent radiologic findings
    REF: Dis. Chest 53:481–486, 1968

20. Gram-negative osteomyelitis may be described by all of the following statements EXCEPT
   A. closed suction irrigation of orthopedic infections with antibiotic solution may be good adjunctive therapy
   B. surgical intervention is seldom necessary if high-dose long-term therapy with appropriate antibiotics is instituted
   C. infections may be clinically indolent, unlike gram-negative pneumonias and bacteremias
   D. surgery or a penetrating wound is an almost invariable antecedent factor in osteomyelitis due to *Pseudomonas*
   E. many patients with acute gram-negative osteomyelitis develop open draining wounds characteristic of chronic disease

   REF: Arch. Intern. Med. 131:228-233, 1973

21. All of the following are true concerning septicemias associated with contaminated intravenous fluids EXCEPT
   A. the single most important therapeutic step is to discontinue the entire IV system, including cannulae or needles
   B. the majority of septicemias related to IV therapy are a result of extrinsic or in-use contamination
   C. organisms associated with intrinsic contamination are frequently sensitive to cephalothin and ampicillin
   D. multiple organisms have been implicated in intrinsic contamination of the same lots of IV solutions
   E. blood cultures should be drawn after removal of the intravenous system

   REF: Morbidity and Mortality Wkly Rpts 22:115-116, 1973

Infectious Diseases

22. All of the statements below correctly describe the shock associated with bacteremia EXCEPT
    A. gram-negative bacillus bacteremia rarely produces shock in patients less than 35 years of age
    B. the pathophysiology is probably the same in shock states induced by gram-negative and gram-positive bacteremias
    C. intra-arterial pressure is an unreliable indicator of the severity of the bacterial shock state
    D. early stages of bacteremic shock evidence hyperventilation, respiratory alkalosis, and an increase in cardiac output
    E. late stages of bacteremic shock evidence perfusion failure, metabolic acidosis, and a decrease in cardiac output
    REF: Medicine 52:287–294, 1973

23. Evaluation of measles vaccine has revealed all of the following EXCEPT
    A. revaccination is necessary in children vaccinated prior to 11 months of age
    B. revaccination is necessary in children who received inactivated vaccine
    C. subclinical reinfection of previously vaccinated children occurs frequently
    D. clinical reinfection of previously vaccinated children is infrequent
    E. the incidence of subacute sclerosing panencephalitis (SSPE) has markedly diminished since introduction of measles vaccine
    REF: Am. J. Epidemiol. 97:365–371, 1973

24. All of the following correctly describe adenovirus infections EXCEPT
    A. they are responsible for a high percentage of acute respiratory infections occurring in hospitalized children
    B. they are responsible for 2%-3% of acute respiratory infections in children ill at home
    C. pleural effusions may occur in up to 14% of children with adenoviral pneumonia
    D. extrapulmonary manifestations are not uncommon in children less than three years old
    E. a significant percentage of patients surviving severe adenoviral pneumonia develop chronic pulmonary diseases
    REF: Am. J. Dis. Child. 126:92-94, 1973

25. Which of the following does NOT describe the nephrotoxicity of amphotericin B?
    A. acute reduction in glomerular filtration rate
    B. defect in urinary acidification with kaliuresis
    C. necrosis of tubular epithelium and calcium deposition
    D. impaired urinary concentrating ability
    E. glomerular arteriolitis
    REF: Semin. Drug Treat. 2:313-329, 1972

26. Which of the statements about ascariasis is INCORRECT?
    A. adults reside in lumen of small bowel
    B. infection results from ingestion of eggs that migrate through lungs as vermicules and mature in small bowel after being swallowed
    C. heavy infestation may result in bowel obstruction
    D. eosinophilia is invariably absent
    E. therapy is with pyratel pamoate, mebendazole, or piperazine
    REF: Maegraith, B.G.: Adams and Maegraith: *Clinical Tropical Diseases, 5th Ed.,* Blackwell Scientific Publications, Oxford and Edinburgh, 1971, pp. 513-515

Infectious Diseases

27. All of the following statements concerning amikacin is correct EXCEPT
   A. amikacin is a recently developed semisynthetic derivative of kanamycin A
   B. amikacin is primarily excreted by glomerular filtration
   C. amikacin is highly bound to serum protein
   D. amikacin's volume of distribution mathematically approximates the extracellular fluid base
   E. amikacin is potentially ototoxic and nephrotoxic
   REF: Clin. Pharmacol. Ther. 15:610–616, 1974
   Antimicrob. Agents Chemother. 3:478–483, 1973
   Antimicrob. Agents Chemother. 9:956–961, 1976
   Ann. Intern. Med. 83:790–800, 1975

28. All of the following statements concerning guidelines for urinary catheters are correct EXCEPT
   A. cleansing of the meatal catheter junction with an antiseptic soap should be done every 72 hours
   B. a sterile closed drainage system should always be used
   C. normal unobstructed downhill flow must be maintained at all times
   D. in patients with urinary catheterization of less than two weeks duration, routine catheter changes are not necessary except when obstruction, contamination, or other malfunctions occur
   E. catheterized patients should be separated from each other whenever possible and should not share the same room or adjacent baths
   REF: Ann. Intern. Med. 82:386–390, 1975

29. All of the following statements concerning the etiology of gastroenteritis in children are correct EXCEPT
    A. bacterial diarrhea appears to occur more commonly in the summer
    B. rotavirus and enteropathic *E. coli* are the most common pathogens in infants
    C. rotavirus and enteropathogenic *E. coli* are the most common pathogens in infants
    D. shigella appears to be the most common pathogen in older children
    E. bacterial pathogens are frequently isolated in more than 90% of children hospitalized with gastroenteritis
    REF: J. Infect. Dis. 136:239–247, 1977

30. All of the following statements concerning odontogenic orofacial infections are correct EXCEPT
    A. obligate anaerobes are recoverable from more than 90% of such patients
    B. 50% of patients have mixed infections containing both aerobes and anaerobes
    C. almost 90% of patients have polymicrobial infection
    D. *Bacteroides, Peptostreptococcus,* and *Streptococcus* are the most prevalent pathogens isolated
    E. mandibular osteomyelitis is rarely if ever due to *Actinomyces*
    REF: Ann. Intern. Med. 88:392–402, 1978

62 / Infectious Diseases

31. All of the following statements concerning tuberculous meningitis in children are correct EXCEPT
   A. tuberculous meningitis commonly has an insidious onset, with gradual or intermittent increases in symptoms
   B. the onset of meningitis in a tuberculous child may be precipitated by measles, head injury, a recent surgical procedure with the patient under general anesthesia, or a severe sunburn
   C. in children with tuberculous meningitis, 93% and 72% of the patients had a positive PPD and positive pulmonary x-ray changes, respectively
   D. up to 50% of patients with tuberculous meningitis may have normal cerebral spinal fluids on admission to the hospital
   E. a cerebral angiography triad of ventricular dilation, narrowing of major vessels at the base, and occlusive disease of medium to small vessels due to tuberculous endarteritis may be seen
   REF: Am. J. Dis. Child. 130:364–367, 1976

32. All of the following statements concerning adenine arabinoside therapy of herpes simplex encephalitis are correct EXCEPT
   A. treatment with adenine arabinoside reduced mortality from 70% to 28%
   B. more than 50% of treated survivors had no or moderately debilitating neurologic sequelae
   C. andenine arabinoside produces severe side effects and permanent drug-induced toxicity
   D. the drug must be given early in the course of infection (before the advent of coma) to have a beneficial effect
   E. the use of adenine arabinoside should be coupled with brain biopsy for specific diagnosis to avoid unnecessary treatment of nonresponsive encephalitides that can mimic herpes simplex
   REF: N. Engl. J. Med. 297:289–294, 1977

Infectious Diseases / 63

33. *Y. enterocolitica* infections are characterized by all of the following EXCEPT
   A. infections with *Y. enterocolitica* and *Y. pseudotuberculosis* are similar
   B. fever is one of the most prominent symptoms
   C. diarrhea and nonspecific abdominal pain are common
   D. local tenderness and pain in the right lower quadrant sometimes leads to operation for suspected appendicitis
   E. when the appendix is removed it is usually gangrenous
   REF: Ann. Intern. Med. 81:458–461, 1974

34. The natural history of urethritis in men includes all of the following EXCEPT
   A. most patients have nongonococcal urethritis
   B. the accuracy of the gram stain reading is close to 98%
   C. patients presenting with nongonococcal urethritis usually have symptoms of dysuria and discharge of short duration
   D. spontaneous purulent discharge is found only in patients with gonococcal urethritis
   E. most patients with nongonococcal urethritis have no discharge or a mucoid discharge obtained only after stripping of the penis
   REF: Ann. Intern. Med. 82:7–12, 1975

35. All of the following statements concerning acute interstitial nephritis due to methicillin are correct EXCEPT
   A. all patients have severe renal dysfunction with an average peak serum creatinine of 8 mg/dl
   B. peripheral eosinophilia is extremely unusual in these patients
   C. all patients have sterile pyuria
   D. many patients have eosinophiliuria determined by examination of urine sediment utilizing Wright's stain
   E. therapy with prednisone appears to be effective in shortening the duration of renal failure in patients with acute interstitial nephritis due to methicillin
   REF: Am. J. Med. 65:756–765, 1978

36. All of the following statements concerning a newly discovered halophilic *Vibrio* species are true EXCEPT
   A. there are two distinct clinical presentations of illness due to this organism, a septicemia form or a wound infection
   B. this new pathogen should be considered in the differential diagnosis of septicemia with secondary skin lesions and of wound infections after exposure to sea water
   C. most cases occur during the winter months without age or sexual predilection
   D. the septicemic form is usually seen in patients with pre-existing hepatic disease who have eaten raw oysters
   E. the wound infections were seen after patients were exposed to sea water or injury occurred during the handling of crabs

   REF: N. Engl. J. Med. 300:1-5, 1979

37. Which one of the following organisms is NOT associated with transmission to man from seafood or shellfish?
   A. a halophilic lactose-fermenting *Vibrio* species
   B. *Campylobacter* (Vibrio) *fetus*
   C. *Vibrio parahemolyticus*
   D. *Vibrio alginolyticus*
   E. *Erysipelothrix insidiosa*

   REF: Ibid.

38. All of the following statements concerning *Chlamydia trachomatis* infections in female college students are correct EXCEPT
   A. cervical infections with *C. trachomatis* can persist for a relatively long period of time
   B. many women infected with *C. trachomatis* are asymptomatic and infected women cannot be differentiated from noninfected women on the basis of symptoms
   C. the natural history of sexually acquired chlamydial infection in women is quite well defined
   D. there is convincing evidence that *C. trachomatis* is a cause of pelvic inflammatory disease
   E. sexual partners of women carrying *C. trachomatis* may contract nongonococcal urethritis, and infants of infected mothers may have conjunctivitis or pneumonia
   REF: N. Engl. J. Med. 300:123-125, 1979

39. Which one of the following diseases is NOT frequently produced by *C. trachomatis*?
   A. nongonococcal urethritis
   B. infantile pneumonia
   C. pelvic inflammatory disease
   D. epididymitis
   E. granuloma inguinale
   REF: Ibid.

40. Which of the following is (are) a diagnostic clue(s) to the presence of factitious or fraudulent fever?
   A. absence of tachycardia in the face of an abrupt rise in body temperature
   B. despite a report of chronic illness, the patient appears well and without any characteristics of illness
   C. the absence of physical or clinical abnormalities along with normal laboratory studies, especially CBC and ESR, in a patient with a true organic fever is unexpected
   D. all patients with fever of undetermined origin should have careful documentation of their fever by observed rectal temperature on several occasions
   E. all of the above
   REF: Am. J. Med. 65:745-755, 1978

41. All of the following statements concerning brain abscesses are true EXCEPT
  A. brain abscesses frequently present as an expanding intracranial lesion with headache and focal neurologic signs rather than as infectious processes
  B. fever is frequently absent
  C. lumbar puncture usually provides useful information
  D. streptococci are the most frequently isolated organisms
  E. brain abscesses showed a peak incidence in the first two decades of life and in the two decades between 50 and 70 years of age
  REF: Ann. Intern. Med. 82:571–576, 1975

42. All of the following statements concerning *Bordetella parapertussis* are correct EXCEPT
  A. *B. parapertussis* is felt to be the etiology of disease in less than 5% of children with clinical pertussis but goes up to 30% in some series
  B. less than 20% of children infected with *B. parapertussis* present with symptoms of clinical pertussis, and approximately 40% are asymptomatic
  C. asymptomatic infections are extremely rare with *B. pertussis*
  D. immunity to *B. pertussis* confers immunity to *B. parapertussis*
  E. *B. parapertussis* may be a major cause of prolonged bronchitis
  REF: Am. J. Dis. Child. 131:560–563, 1977

43. Whipple's disease is an infrequently occurring condition characterized by weight loss, diarrhea, arthralgia, and abdominal pain. All of the following statements concerning Whipple's disease are correct EXCEPT

A. biopsies of small intestine mucosa and/or lymph nodes have become practical and reliable sources for establishing the diagnosis of Whipple's disease

B. tissues involved in Whipple's disease show large numbers of foamy macrophages with abundant cytoplasm containing clumped periodic acid-Schiff (PAS)-positive, diastase-resistant material

C. electron microscopic studies show bacilliform structures within macrophages in tissues of patients with Whipple's disease

D. bacilliform structures in PAS-positive macrophages have not been found in patients with Whipple's disease outside the GI tract and lymph nodes

E. Whipple's disease is amenable to curative therapy with antibiotics

REF: Am. J. Med. 65:873–880, 1978

44. Which of the following statements regarding herpes zoster is NOT correct?

A. zoster occurs throughout the year without seasonal predominance

B. it occurs most frequently in association with lymphoproliferative malignancies

C. lesions are usually confined to the skin in one or more adjacent dermatomes and are most frequent in the thoracic region

D. predisposing factors for zoster include local irradiation and occasionally surgery in subsequently involved areas

E. advanced stages of Hodgkin's disease are associated with an increased incidence of zoster

REF: Am. J. Med. 65:738–743, 1978

45. All of the following statements concerning covert bacteriuria in schoolgirls are correct EXCEPT
   A. treatment of covert bacteriuria in girls aged five to 12 had no effect on the emergence of symptoms
   B. treatment had no effect on the clearance of vesicoureteric reflux
   C. screening for covert bacteriuria is recommended, since kidney damage can be prevented by therapy
   D. three-quarters of treated girls but only one-quarter of untreated controls were free of infection for at least half of a four-year follow-up
   E. new kidney scars do not develop in previously unscarred kidneys in females with covert bacteriuria
   REF: Lancet I:889–893, 1978

46. All of the following intestinal pathogens usually have been associated with venereal transmission and symptomatic illness in homosexuals EXCEPT
   A. shigellosis
   B. giardiasis
   C. amebiasis
   D. hepatitis
   E. brucellosis
   REF: J.A.M.A. 238:1386–1387, 1978
         Br. J. Vener. Dis. 52:348–350, 1976

47. Cefazolin can be used safely and successfully in the treatment of infections due to all of the following organisms EXCEPT
   A. *S. aureus*
   B. Group A and Group B streptococci
   C. *S. pneumoniae*
   D. nonenterococcal Group D streptococci
   E. enterococcal Group D streptococci
   REF: Ann. Intern. Med. 89 (part 1):650–656, 1978

48. Ludwig's angina was first described in 1836 by von Ludwig and is characterized correctly by all of the following statements EXCEPT
   A. is invariably caused by a mixed bacterial infection composed of staphylococci and streptococci
   B. is a rapidly spreading gangrenous cellulitis or phlegma involving both the submaxillary and sublingual spaces
   C. pathogenesis is usually related to precipitating factors within the oral cavity such as dental infections, foreign bodies, lacerations of the floor of the mouth, and other maxillofacial injuries
   D. an understanding of the potential spaces defined by the deep cervical fascia is essential to the therapeutic approach
   E. therapy must include the provision of an adequate airway, usually in the form of a tracheotomy
   REF: J. Oral Surg. 34:456–460, 1976
   Am. J. Med. 53:257–260, 1972

49. All of the following questions concerning gastroenteritis in children are correct EXCEPT
   A. reovirus-like agents have been detected in fecal extracts of infants and young children with acute gastroenteritis in many parts of the world
   B. reoviruses are rarely detected in children over the age of six
   C. reoviruses are more often encountered in winter than in summer as causes of gastroenteritis
   D. electrophoretic patterns of viral RNA suggest that there are at least two different reovirus-like agents associated with infantile gastroenteritis
   E. two different reoviruses are responsible for infantile gastroenteritis and epidemic gastroenteritis of children respectively
   REF: J. Clin. Microbiol. 6:502–506, 1977
   Am. J. Epidemiol. 197:161–169, 1978

50. Which of the following statements concerning infections with *Eikenella corrodens*, a newly recognized human pathogen, is NOT true?
   A. *E. corrodens* is a facultative anaerobic gram-negative bacillus
   B. *E. corrodens* is a frequent inhabitant of the upper respiratory tract
   C. this organism can be isolated from the gastrointestinal and genitourinary tracts
   D. advanced age, ruptured viscus, and underlying carcinoma seemed to antedate most infection with this organism
   E. *E. corrodens* is usually sensitive to clindamycin
   REF: Ann. Intern. Med. 80:305–309, 1974

51. The diagnosis of clindamycin-associated diarrhea is best established by which one of the following?
   A. abdominal cramps
   B. mucoid diarrhea
   C. bloody diarrhea
   D. edema of the bowel present on proctoscopic examination
   E. presence of pseudomembrane on proctoscopic examination
   REF: Ann. Intern. Med. 81:429–433, 1974

52. Each statement about strongyloidiasis is correct EXCEPT
   A. embryonated eggs may usually be seen in duodenal aspirates
   B. rhabditiform larvae may be seen in duodenal aspirates
   C. embyronated eggs are not usually seen in stool specimens
   D. filariform larvae are not seen in stool specimens
   E. rhabditiform larvae are often seen in stool specimens
   REF: Medicine 57:427–544, 1978

53. All of the following statements concerning *Haemophilus influenzae* meningitis in children are correct EXCEPT
    A. there is no difference in mortality in patients treated with chloramphenicol versus ampicillin
    B. complete recovery without handicapping sequelae occurs in approximately 60% of patients
    C. children treated with chloramphenicol have significantly fewer eighth nerve defects than those treated with ampicillin
    D. seizure disorders are a sequel of *H. influenzae* in approximately 7% of patients
    E. subdural fusions occur predominantly in those patients under two years of age
    REF: Acta Paediatr. Scand. 67:17-24, 1978

54. All of the following statements concerning *P. carinii* pneumonia are correct EXCEPT
    A. *P. carinii* is probably acquired by the respiratory route
    B. specific serologic tests of high sensitivity for antipneumocystis antibodies make it possible to diagnose infection and to identify potential carriers
    C. pneumocystis attack rates are higher in patients who receive more intensive antileukemic therapy
    D. acquisition and spread of pneumocystis may be related to contact of immunosuppressed patients with factors in the hospital environment
    E. *P. carinii* is a well-known cause of epidemic interstitial pneumonia in premature and debilitated infants
    REF: Am. J. Dis. Child. 132:143-148, 1978

55. All of the following statements concerning septic pulmonary embolization are correct EXCEPT
    A. the incidence is high following suppurative pelvic thrombophlebitis
    B. it most commonly results from primary right-sided endocarditis
    C. signs and symptoms may include dyspnea, tachypnea, chest pain, tachycardia, cough, hemoptysis, restlessness, anxiety, and syncope along with shaking chills and high fever
    D. roentgenographic findings are helpful but often subtle and may be characterized by small parenchymal densities as the only suggestion of this diagnosis
    E. *S. aureus* is the most common offending organism in all patient populations, except for the patient with thermal injury in which gram-negative organisms predominate
    REF: Surg. Gynecol. Obstet. 144:105–108, 1977

56. All of the following cardiac lesions are sufficiently susceptible to the development of endocarditis from transient bacteremia to unequivocally warrant the use of antimicrobial prophylaxis during dental manipulations or genitourinary or abdominal procedures EXCEPT
    A. tetralogy of Fallot
    B. ventricular septal defect
    C. atrial septal defect, secundum type
    D. patent ductus arteriosus
    E. valvular aortic stenosis
    REF: Circulation 51:581–588, 1975

Infectious Diseases / 73

57. All of the following statements concerning initial empiric therapy in patients with severe sepsis of intra-abdominal, soft tissue, female genital, or oral pulmonary origin are correct EXCEPT
 A. Group D streptococci are one of the most frequent organisms isolated from infections of this nature
 B. a combination of clindamycin and gentamicin appears to be highly effective prospective therapy
 C. surgical intervention combined with antimicrobial therapy appears more effective than antimicrobial therapy alone
 D. obligate anaerobes in addition to aerobes are extremely important in serious infections of abdominal, soft tissue, female genital, or oral pulmonary origin
 E. clindamycin-associated pseudomembranous colitis does not occur frequently enough to obviate its use in this situation
 REF: Can. Med. Assoc. J. 115:1225-1229, 1976

58. Each of the following organisms is an etiologic agent of hospital-acquired deep fungus infection EXCEPT
 A. *Torulopsis glabrata*
 B. *Geotrichum candidum*
 C. *Cryptococcus neoformans*
 D. *Blastomyces dermatitidis*
 E. *Actinomyces israelii*
 REF: Medicine 54:499-507, 1975

59. All of the following statements concerning deep mycotic infection in the hospitalized adult are true EXCEPT
   A. *Candida* species are the most common organisms producing deep mycotic infection in the hospitalized patient
   B. almost all patients with *Candida* infection have significant underlying disease
   C. the most common portal of entry for systemic *Candida* infection is through the venous catheter
   D. the most common predisposing therapy to deep candidal infection is the use of broad-spectrum antimicrobial agents
   E. systemic candidal infection is easily diagnosed and successfully treated
   REF: Ibid.

60. Features that help to distinguish Legionnaires' disease from viral pneumonia include all of the following EXCEPT
   A. the extent of hypoxemia
   B. elevated leukocyte counts
   C. renal involvement
   D. central nervous system involvement
   E. both renal and central nervous involvement
   REF: Ann. Intern. Med. 88:294-302, 1978

61. All of the following are predisposing factors to *S. aureus* sternal osteomyelitis EXCEPT
   A. bone marrow aspiration
   B. prior trauma to the sternum
   C. intravenous drug use
   D. leukemia
   E. median sternotomy surgical incisions
   REF: So. Med. J. 71:348-349, 1978

62. To date, antibiotic combinations have been widely prescribed for a variety of purposes. Each of the following is a correct current purpose of the use of antimicrobial combinations EXCEPT
   A. to achieve broad antimicrobial activity in critically ill patients with undefined bacterial infection
   B. to treat mixed bacterial infections, the components of which may not have a common antibiotic susceptibility
   C. to prevent the emergence of resistance against the single antibiotic
   D. to achieve an additive or synergistic effect against a single organism
   E. to reduce the toxicity of one agent through the use of another
   REF: Medicine 57:179-195, 1978

63. Systemic prophylactic antibiotics have been demonstrated to be effective in reducing postoperative infection in all of the following surgical procedures EXCEPT
   A. vaginal hysterectomy
   B. cesarean section
   C. exploratory laparotomy
   D. Charnley total hip operations
   E. microsurgical craniotomies
   REF: Arch. Surg. 112:326-333, 1977

V: Endocrinology

DIRECTIONS: Each of the questions or incomplete statements below is followed by five suggested answers or completions. Select the **one** that is BEST in each case.

I. Hypothalamus and Pituitary

1. The most common cause of hypopituitarism in the adult is
   A. allergic hypophysitis
   B. pituitary adenoma
   C. craniopharyngioma
   D. pituitary infarction
   E. pituitary sarcoidosis
   REF: Williams, R.H. (Ed): *Textbook of Endocrinology, 5th Ed.*, W.B. Saunders Company, Philadelphia, 1974, pp. 55-56
   Beeson, P.B., McDermott, W., Wyngaarden, J.B. (Eds): *Cecil Textbook of Medicine, 15th Ed.*, W.B. Saunders Company, Philadelphia, 1979, pp. 2100-2102

Endocrinology

2. The earliest clinical complaint in an adult man with a destructive lesion of the pituitary fossa is likely to be
   A. dry skin and cold intolerance
   B. impotence
   C. postural faintness
   D. tremor and sweating, relieved by eating
   E. skin pallor
   REF: Williams, R.H. (Ed): *Textbook of Endocrinology, 5th Ed.*, W.B. Saunders Company, Philadelphia, 1974, pp. 56-58
   Bondy, P.K. and Rosenberg, L.E. (Eds): *Duncan's Diseases of Metabolism, 8th Ed.*, W.B. Saunders Company, Philadelphia, 1979, pp. 990-992
   Beeson, P.B., McDermott, W., Wyngaarden, J.B. (Eds): *Cecil Textbook of Medicine, 15th Ed.*, W.B. Saunders Company, Philadelphia, 1979, pp. 2100-2103

3. The cranial nerve most frequently damaged by an expanding pituitary tumor is
   A. I
   B. II
   C. III
   D. IV
   E. VI
   REF: Williams, R.H. (Ed): *Textbook of Endocrinology, 5th Ed.*, W.B. Saunders Company, Philadelphia, 1974, p. 68

4. The most reliable method for diagnosing active acromegaly is
   A. measurement of the serum phosphorus
   B. examination of skull x-rays
   C. examination of hand x-rays
   D. serial measurement of growth hormone before and after administration of insulin
   E. serial measurement of growth hormone before and after administration of glucose
   REF: Ibid., p. 73

5. The test most likely to be of diagnostic value in a 25-year-old woman with persistent nonpuerperal galactorrhea and amenorrhea is
   A. x-rays of the sella turcica
   B. serum estrogen level
   C. serum LH level
   D. serum prolactin level
   E. endometrial biopsy
   REF: Bondy, P.K. and Rosenberg, L.E. (Eds): *Duncan's Diseases of Metabolism, 8th Ed.,* W.B. Saunders Company, Philadelphia, 1979, p. 1000

6. The most consistent diagnostic finding in patients with Cushing's disease (pituitary ACTH overproduction) is
   A. x-ray enlargement of the sella turcica
   B. failure to suppress ACTH production with large doses of glucocorticoids (e.g., 8 mg dexamethasone per day)
   C. suppression of ACTH production with large doses of glucocorticoids, but not with smaller doses that would be suppressive in normal subjects (e.g., 2 mg dexamethasone per day)
   D. failure to increase ACTH production by administration of metyrapone
   E. decreased response of the adrenals to a test dose of ACTH
   REF: Williams, R.H. (Ed): *Textbook of Endocrinology, 5th Ed.,* W.B. Saunders Company, Philadelphia, 1974, pp. 258-261
   Beeson, P.B., McDermott, W., Wyngaarden, J.B. (Eds): *Cecil Textbook of Medicine, 15th Ed.,* W.B. Saunders Company, Philadelphia, 1979, pp. 2154, 2155

DIRECTIONS: For each of the following questions or incomplete statements ONE or MORE of the answers or completions given is correct. Select:
    A if only 1, 2 and 3 are correct,
    B if only 1 and 3 are correct,
    C if only 2 and 4 are correct,
    D if only 4 is correct,
    E if all are correct.

7. A patient with a destructive lesion in the medial basal hypothalamus would be likely to show
   1. decreased growth hormone secretory response to hypoglycemia
   2. decreased cortisol response to hypoglycemia
   3. decreased serum gonadotropins
   4. decreased serum prolactin
   REF: Beeson, P.B., McDermott, W., Wyngaarden, J.B. (Eds): *Cecil Textbook of Medicine, 15th Ed.,* W.B.Saunders Company, Philadelphia, 1979, pp. 2078-2082

8. A patient with Sheehan's syndrome (postpartum pituitary necrosis) would be likely to show
   1. decreased secretion of gonadotropins
   2. decreased secretion of prolactin
   3. decreased secretion of growth hormone
   4. decreased secretion of vasopressin
   REF: Williams, R.H. (Ed): *Textbook of Endocrinology, 5th Ed.,* W.B. Saunders Company, Philadelphia, 1974, pp. 55-56
   Bondy, P.K. and Rosenberg, L.E. (Eds): *Duncan's Diseases of Metabolism, 8th Ed.,* W.B. Saunders Company, Philadelphia, 1979, p. 988

9. Which of the following is a typical finding in a patient with the empty sella syndrome?
   1. hypogonadism
   2. hypothyroidism
   3. diabetes insipidus
   4. radiological evidence of enlargement of the sella turcica
   REF: Bondy, P.K. and Rosenberg, L.E. (Eds): *Duncan's Diseases of Metabolism, 8th Ed.,* W.B. Saunders Company, Philadelphia, 1979, p. 1003

10. The clinical uses of thyrotropin-releasing hormone (TRH) include
    1. treatment of patients with myxedema
    2. testing the pituitary for ability to secrete thyroid-stimulating hormone (TSH)
    3. testing the functional reserve of the thyroid gland
    4. testing the pituitary for ability to secrete prolactin
    REF: Beeson, P.B., McDermott, W., Wyngaarden, J.B. (Eds): *Cecil Textbook of Medicine, 15th Ed.,* W.B. Saunders Company, Philadelphia, 1979, pp. 2081-2119

11. Potential clinical uses for the drug bromocriptine include
    1. suppression of prolactin secretion by pituitary tumors
    2. suppression of ACTH secretion in patients with Cushing's disease
    3. suppression of growth hormone secretion in patients with acromegaly
    4. suppression of gonadotropin secretion in women who do not wish to take an estrogen-containing oral contraceptive
    REF: Thorner, et al.: Brit. Med. J. 1:299-303, 1975
          Jacobs: N. Engl. J. Med. 295:954-956, 1976

12. Anorexia nervosa usually differs from hypopituitarism, since in anorexia nervosa
    1. serum growth hormone is not low
    2. serum luteinizing hormone (LH) and follicle-stimulating hormone (FSH) are not low
    3. serum cortisol is not low
    4. serum T_3 (by radioimmunoassay) is not low
    REF: Williams, R.H. (Ed): *Textbook of Endocrinology, 5th Ed.,* W.B. Saunders Company, Philadelphia, 1974, p. 58

Directions Summarized				
A	B	C	D	E
1, 2, 3 only	1, 3 only	2, 4 only	4 only	All are correct

13. The clinical diagnosis of diabetes insipidus requires the demonstration of
    1. a destructive lesion in the region of the hypothalamus
    2. urine osmolality remains inappropriately low in the presence of an elevated serum osmolality
    3. immunoreactive vasopressin from plasma
    4. kidney response to exogenous vasopressin by production of more concentrated urine
    REF: Ibid., p. 87

14. The hyponatremia often seen in patients with hypopituitarism is a result of
    1. cortisol deficiency
    2. aldosterone deficiency
    3. water retention with dilution of extracellular sodium
    4. excessive urinary sodium loss
    REF: Beeson, P.B., McDermott, W., Wyngaarden, J.B. (Eds): *Cecil Textbook of Medicine, 15th Ed.,* W.B. Saunders Company, Philadelphia, 1979, p. 2101

15. The syndrome of inappropriate secretion of antidiuretic hormone (SIADH) should be suspected in a patient with
    1. hyponatremia, edema, and elevated plasma aldosterone
    2. hyponatremia, hyperkalemia, and weight loss
    3. hyponatremia, urine osmolality of 100 mOsm/L
    4. hyponatremia, urine osmolality of 600 mOsm/L
    REF: Williams, R.H. (Ed): *Textbook of Endocrinology, 5th Ed.,* W.B. Saunders Company, Philadelphia, 1974, p. 91

16. Appropriate therapy for a patient with SIADH might include
    1. increased dietary intake of sodium
    2. restricted intake of water
    3. administration of 9-α-fluorocortisol
    4. administration of demeclocycline
    REF: Ibid.

DIRECTIONS: Each of the questions or incomplete statements below is followed by suggested answers or completions. Select the **one** that is **BEST** in each case.

II. Adrenal Cortex and Medulla

17. The most important factor governing rapid physiologic adjustments in aldosterone secretion is
    A. angiotensinogen
    B. angiotensin I
    C. angiotensin II
    D. serum potassium concentration
    E. ACTH
    REF: Williams, R.H. (Ed): *Textbook of Endocrinology, 5th Ed.*, W.B. Saunders Company, Philadelphia, 1974, pp. 211-212, 948-949

18. The diagnosis of Addison's disease can be made with certainty when
    A. plasma cortisol is less than 8 μg/100 ml
    B. the combination of hyponatremia and hyperkalemia is present
    C. plasma ACTH is found to be elevated in a patient with previously unexplained hypotension
    D. urinary 17-hydroxysteroids are less than 10 mg per 24 hours (8 mg/gm of urinary creatinine) and fail to rise after repeated ACTH infusion
    REF: Ibid., p. 273
    Bondy, P.K. and Rosenberg, L.E. (Eds): *Duncan's Diseases of Metabolism, 8th Ed.*, W.B. Saunders Company, Philadelphia, 1979, pp. 1136-1137

84 / Endocrinology

19. A patient whose urinary 17-hydroxysteroid output is suppressed on a 8.0 mg per day dose of dexamethasone but not by 2.0 mg per day probably has
   A. an adrenal cortical tumor
   B. pituitary ACTH excess (Cushing's disease)
   C. ectopic overproduction of ACTH by a nonpituitary neoplasm
   D. a form of congenital adrenal hyperplasia
   E. a normal pituitary adrenal axis
   REF: Williams, R.H. (Ed): *Textbook of Endocrinology, 5th Ed.,* W.B. Saunders Company, Philadelphia, 1974, pp. 251-261
   Bondy, P.K. and Rosenberg, L.E. (Eds): *Duncan's Diseases of Metabolism, 8th Ed.,* W.B. Saunders Company, Philadelphia, 1979, p. 1147

20. A virilized 18-year-old woman is found to have baseline urinary 17-hydroxysteroids of 10 mg and 17-ketosteroids of 35 mg per 24 hours. After 3 days of dexamethasone (2.0 mg/day), the 17-hydroxysteroids are 2 mg, and the 17-ketosteroids 5 mg per 24 hours. The most likely diagnosis is
   A. idiopathic hirsutism
   B. adrenal carcinoma
   C. ovarian carcinoma
   D. Cushing's syndrome
   E. adrenogenital syndrome due to a biosynthetic defect in cortisol production
   REF: Williams, R.H. (Ed): *Textbook of Endocrinology, 5th Ed.,* W.B. Saunders Company, Philadelphia, 1974, pp. 247, 276-279
   Beeson, P.B., McDermott, W., Wyngaarden, J.B. (Eds): *Cecil Textbook of Medicine, 15th Ed.,* W.B. Saunders Company, Philadelphia, 1979, pp. 2158-2162

21. The best screening test for the diagnosis of pheochromocytoma is
    A. measurement of blood pressure before and after the administration of phentolamine
    B. measurement of blood pressure before and after the administration of histamine
    C. measurement of plasma catecholamines
    D. measurement of 24-hour urinary metanephrines
    E. bilateral adrenal angiography
    REF: Williams, R.H. (Ed): *Textbook of Endocrinology, 5th Ed.,* W.B. Saunders Company, Philadelphia, 1974, p. 310
    Bondy, P.K. and Rosenberg, L.E. (Eds): *Duncan's Diseases of Metabolism, 8th Ed.,* W.B. Saunders Company, Philadelphia, 1979, pp. 1208-1209

DIRECTIONS: For each of the following questions or incomplete statements, **ONE** or **MORE** of the answers or completions given is correct. Select:
   A if only 1, 2 and 3 are correct,
   B if only 1 and 3 are correct,
   C if only 2 and 4 are correct,
   D if only 4 is correct,
   E if all are correct.

---

22. In the normal subject, levels of plasma cortisol are influenced by
    1. the time of day, with higher levels early in the morning
    2. acute stress such as trauma or infection
    3. recent use of glucocorticoid drugs
    4. ingestion of a carbohydrate-rich meal
    REF: Williams, R.H. (Ed): *Textbook of Endocrinology, 5th Ed.,* W.B. Saunders Company, Philadelphia, 1974, pp. 239-240

Directions Summarized

A	B	C	D	E
1, 2, 3 only	1, 3 only	2, 4 only	4 only	All are correct

23. Iatrogenic Cushing's syndrome
    1. is usually associated with limited pituitary ACTH reserve
    2. may be avoided by selecting a synthetic glucocorticoid with very high anti-inflammatory activity
    3. may be ameliorated by administering the total steroid dose required over a 48-hour period as a single dose every second morning
    4. is less common than spontaneous Cushing's syndrome
    REF: Ibid., p. 281
    >   Bondy, P.K. and Rosenberg, L.E. (Eds): *Duncan's Diseases of Metabolism, 8th Ed.,* W.B. Saunders Company, Philadelphia, 1979, p. 1156

24. Adrenal cortical carcinoma
    1. is usually discovered because of its tendency to overproduce glucocorticoids, androgens, or estrogens
    2. is strongly suggested by the findings of very high urinary 17-hydroxysteroids or 17-ketosteroids and low plasma ACTH
    3. tends to invade neighboring organs such as the inferior vena cava and liver in the majority of cases before a correct diagnosis is made
    4. may be treated with the adrenocorticolytic drug, o-p'-DDD for palliative chemotherapy
    REF: Williams, R.H. (Ed): *Textbook of Endocrinology, 5th Ed.,* W.B. Saunders Company, Philadelphia, 1974, pp. 258-260, 270

Endocrinology / 87

25. A patient with hypertension due to primary hyperaldosteronism would be expected to show
   1. inappropriately elevated plasma aldosterone after salt loading
   2. inappropriately suppressed plasma renin activity after sodium depletion
   3. serum potassium less than 4.0 mEq/L
   4. a fall in blood pressure after therapy with spironolactone
   REF: Ibid., pp. 267-268
   Beeson, P.B., McDermott, W., Wyngaarden, J.B. (Eds): *Cecil Textbook of Medicine, 15th Ed.,* W.B. Saunders Company, Philadelphia, 1979, pp. 2157-2158

26. In which forms of hypertension listed below would the plasma renin activity usually be elevated?
   1. essential hypertension
   2. malignant hypertension
   3. hypertension secondary to Cushing's syndrome
   4. hypertension due to renal artery stenosis
   REF: Williams, R.H. (Ed): *Textbook of Endocrinology, 5th Ed.,* W.B. Saunders Company, Philadelphia, 1974, pp. 952-961

27. Patients with primary and secondary adrenal insufficiency can be differentiated by
   1. demonstrating that the urinary 17-hydroxysteroids rise after administration of ACTH, but not after administration of metyrapone
   2. demonstrating that plasma cortisol fails to rise after metyrapone
   3. demonstrating that plasma ACTH fails to rise after metyrapone
   4. demonstrating that plasma cortisol fails to rise after a single intravenous dose of ACTH
   REF: Ibid., pp. 251, 270-271
   Bondy, P.K. and Rosenberg, L.E. (Eds): *Duncan's Diseases of Metabolism, 8th Ed.,* W.B. Saunders Company, Philadelphia, 1979, pp. 1137, 1142-1143

Directions Summarized				
A	B	C	D	E
1, 2, 3 only	1, 3 only	2, 4 only	4 only	All are correct

28. Pheochromocytomas are
    1. unilateral in about 90% of cases
    2. benign in about 90% of cases
    3. more likely to be multifocal in familial cases than in sporadic cases
    4. most often found adjacent to the abdominal aorta when they occur in extra-adrenal sites
    REF: Williams, R.H. (Ed): *Textbook of Endocrinology, 5th Ed.*, W.B. Saunders Company, Philadelphia, 1974, p. 307
    Bondy, P.K. and Rosenberg, L.E. (Eds): *Duncan's Diseases of Metabolism, 8th Ed.*, W.B. Saunders Company, Philadelphia, 1979, pp. 1204-1207

DIRECTIONS: Each of the questions or incomplete statements below is followed by five suggested answers or completions. Select the **one** that is **BEST** in each case.

III. Thyroid

29. The most sensitive laboratory test for the detection of primary thyroid failure is
    A. serum cholesterol
    B. serum T_4
    C. serum T_3 (radioimmunoassay RIA)
    D. serum TSH
    E. serum T_3 resin uptake
    REF: Williams, R.H. (Ed): *Textbook of Endocrinology, 5th Ed.*, W.B. Saunders Company, Philadelphia, 1974, p. 146

30. The thyrotoxicosis of Graves' disease is probably caused by
    A. an autonomous hyperfunctioning thyroid adenoma
    B. overproduction of TSH
    C. an antibody that binds to the TSH receptor to cause thyroid stimulation
    D. excess ingestion of iodides
    E. viral infection of the thyroid
    REF: Ibid., pp. 163-165
    Bondy, P.K. and Rosenberg, L.E. (Eds): *Duncan's Diseases of Metabolism, 8th Ed.,* W. B. Saunders Company, Philadelphia, 1979, p. 1069
    Beeson, P.B., McDermott, W., Wyngaarden, J.B. (Eds): *Cecil Textbook of Medicine, 15th Ed.,* W.B. Saunders Company, Philadelphia, 1979, pp. 2120-2121

31. A drug that can reverse the symptoms of thyrotoxicosis without reducing the secretion of thyroid hormones by the thyroid gland is
    A. propylthiouracil
    B. lithium carbonate
    C. potassium iodide
    D. radioactive iodine
    E. propranolol
    REF: Williams, R.H. (Ed): *Textbook of Endocrinology, 5th Ed.,* W.B. Saunders Company Philadelphia, 1974, pp. 182-183
    Beeson, P.B., McDermott, W., Wyngaarden, J.B. (Eds): *Cecil Textbook of Medicine, 15th Ed.,* W.B. Saunders Company, Philadelphia, 1979, pp. 2123-2125

DIRECTIONS: Each of the questions or incomplete statements below is followed by five suggested answers or completions. Select the **one** that is **BEST** in each case.

32. The incidence of hypothyroidism after radioactive iodine therapy
    A. is less than 10%
    B. does not show any increase beyond the first five years following treatment
    C. may be reduced to zero by giving just enough ^{131}I to cure the thyrotoxicosis
    D. increases progressively by 2% to 3% for each year following treatment
    E. is higher in patients with toxic multinodular goiters than in patients with Graves' disease
    REF: Williams, R.H. (Ed): *Textbook of Endocrinology, 5th Ed.,* W.B. Saunders Company, Philadelphia, 1974, p. 181
    Bondy, P.K. and Rosenberg, L.E. (Eds): *Duncan's Diseases of Metabolism, 8th Ed.,* W.B. Saunders Company, Philadelphia, 1979, pp. 1074-1075
    Beeson, P.B., McDermott, W., Wyngaarden, J.B. (Eds): *Cecil Textbook of Medicine, 15th Ed.,* W.B. Saunders Company, Philadelphia, 1979, pp. 2124-2125

DIRECTIONS: For each of the following questions or incomplete statements **ONE** or **MORE** of the answers or completions given is correct. Select:
   A if only 1, 2 and 3 are correct,
   B if only 1 and 3 are correct,
   C if only 2 and 4 are correct,
   D if only 4 is correct,
   E if all are correct.

33. Which of the thyroid function tests listed below would be affected by recent intravenous pyelography?
    1. serum T_4 by RIA
    2. serum TSH
    3. serum T_3 resin uptake
    4. thyroidal ^{131}I uptake
    REF: Williams, R.H. (Ed): *Textbook of Endocrinology, 5th Ed.,* W.B. Saunders Company, Philadelphia, 1974, pp. 132-133, 138, 144

34. Which of the thyroid function tests listed below would be affected by the administration of an estrogen-containing oral contraceptive?
    1. serum T_4 (RIA)
    2. serum TSH
    3. serum T_3 resin uptake
    4. thyroidal ^{131}I uptake
    REF: Ibid.

35. Secondary hypothyroidism (due to pituitary failure) can be differentiated from primary hypothyroidism by measuring
    1. serum T_4
    2. serum TSH
    3. thyroid ^{131}I uptake
    4. serum TSH response to TRH
    REF: Ibid., pp. 146-148, 202-203

Directions Summarized				
A	B	C	D	E
1, 2, 3 only	1, 3 only	2, 4 only	4 only	All are correct

36. A normal subject has received 0.2 mg of levothyroxine for the past year. Thyroid function tests would show
   1. normal or slightly elevated serum T_4
   2. absent serum T_3 (RIA)
   3. decreased TSH response to TRH
   4. normal thyroidal uptake of ^{131}I
   REF: Ibid., pp. 208-209
   　　　Beeson, P.B., McDermott, W., Wyngaarden, J.B. (Eds): *Cecil Textbook of Medicine, 15th Ed.*, W.B. Saunders Company, Philadelphia, 1979, pp. 2116-2118

37. Subacute thyroiditis is usually associated with
   1. pain and tenderness of the thyroid gland
   2. hypothyroidism
   3. reduced thyroidal uptake of ^{131}I
   4. elevated antithyroglobulin antibodies
   REF: Williams, R.H. (Ed): *Textbook of Endocrinology, 5th Ed.*, W.B. Saunders Company, Philadelphia, 1974, pp. 187-188
   　　　Beeson, P.B., McDermott, W., Wyngaarden, J.B. (Eds): *Cecil Textbook of Medicine, 15th Ed.*, W.B. Saunders Company, Philadelphia, 1979, pp. 2131-2132

38. Clinical feature(s) that increase the odds of a thyroid nodule being malignant is (are)
    1. generalized enlargement of the entire thyroid gland
    2. hyperfunction of the nodule on a thyroid scintiscan
    3. acute history of pain and enlargement of the nodule
    4. previous history of head or neck irradiation
    REF: Williams, R.H. (Ed): *Textbook of Endocrinology, 5th Ed.*, W.B. Saunders Company, Philadelphia, 1974, pp. 216-222
    Beeson, P.B., McDermott, W., Wyngaarden, J.B. (Eds): *Cecil Textbook of Medicine, 15th Ed.*, W.B. Saunders Company Philadelphia, 1979, pp. 2141-2143

DIRECTIONS: Each of the questions or incomplete statements below is followed by five suggested answers or completions. Select the **one** that is **BEST** in each case.

IV. Ovary and Testis

39. A 35-year-old woman presents with a six-month history of amenorrhea, hirsutism, acne, and clitoromegaly. Urinary 17-ketosteroids are 12 mg/24 hours (normal), plasma testosterone is 400 ng/dl. The right ovary is enlarged. The most likely diagnosis is
    A. idiopathic hirsutism
    B. congenital adrenal hyperplasia
    C. adrenal cortical tumor
    D. ovarian tumor
    E. polycystic ovarian disease
    REF: Williams, R.H. (Ed): *Textbook of Endocrinology, 5th Ed.*, W.B. Saunders Company, Philadelphia, 1974, p. 394

DIRECTIONS: Each of the questions or incomplete statements below is followed by five suggested answers or completions. Select the **one** that is **BEST** in each case.

40. A 23-year-old woman has had amenorrhea for two years. Her menarche occurred at 14½ years, and her menstrual periods were infrequent, scanty, and irregular for the first two years, but then became normal. At age 19, she was diagnosed as having Addison's disease and was begun on cortisol replacement. On physical examination her vaginal mucosa was erythematous and atrophic. Vaginal cytology showed markedly reduced cornification with increased numbers of basal and parabasal cells. Plasma LH was markedly elevated. From the information given the most likely diagnosis is
    A. gonadal dysgenesis
    B. polycystic ovarian disease
    C. psychogenic amenorrhea
    D. "autoimmune" primary ovarian failure
    E. pituitary adenoma
    REF: Ibid., pp. 408-409

41. An adult male presenting with infertility, azoospermia, slightly small testes of normal consistency, normal karyotype, normal testosterone and LH, and high serum FSH probably has
    A. Leydig cell aplasia
    B. Sertoli cell aplasia
    C. germinal cell aplasia ("Sertoli-cell-only-syndrome")
    D. Klinefelter's syndrome
    E. bilateral varicoceles
    REF: Ibid., pp. 341-342

42. A normally developed 18-year-old woman had menarche at age 14 and a pregnancy terminated by therapeutic abortion at age 16. Since then she has been amenorrheic. Following the administration of a single dose of progesterone she fails to have menses. She also fails to bleed after a three-week course of estrogen. The most likely problem is
   A. Turner's syndrome
   B. testicular feminization
   C. pituitary tumor with secondary hypopituitarism
   D. an abnormality of the endometrium
   E. premature menopause
   REF: Ibid., p. 407

DIRECTIONS: For each of the following questions or incomplete statements, **ONE** or **MORE** of the answers or completions given is correct. Select:
   A if only 1, 2 and 3 are correct,
   B if only 1 and 3 are correct,
   C if only 2 and 4 are correct,
   D if only 4 is correct,
   E if all are correct.

---

43. Ovulation in the normal woman
   1. is preceded by an increase in serum LH levels
   2. is preceded by an increase in serum progesterone
   3. is preceded by an increased responsiveness of pituitary LH to the administration of LHRH
   4. is preceded by a fall in serum estrogens
   REF: Beeson, P.B., McDermott, W., Wyngaarden, J.B. (Eds): *Cecil Textbook of Medicine, 15th Ed.*, W.B. Saunders Company, Philadelphia, 1979, pp. 2175-2179

Directions Summarized				
A	B	C	D	E
1, 2, 3 only	1, 3 only	2, 4 only	4 only	All are correct

44. Normal menopause is preceded by
    1. reduced serum estradiol levels
    2. elevated serum levels of LH and FSH
    3. reduced serum progesterone levels
    4. reduced pituitary LH response to LHRH
    REF: Williams, R.H. (Ed): *Textbook of Endocrinology, 5th Ed.,* W.B. Saunders Company, Philadelphia, 1974, p. 390

45. As males enter the sixth and seventh decades of life, one commonly finds
    1. a decrease in testicular size
    2. a decrease in testosterone secretion rates
    3. subnormal levels of plasma testosterone
    4. a gradual decline in libido and sexual activity
    REF: Ibid., pp. 346-347

46. Administration of exogenous androgens is likely to relieve symptoms of decreased libido and sexual potential in males with
    1. psychogenic impotence
    2. diabetic autonomic neuropathy
    3. Leriche's syndrome
    4. testicular damage due to a prior attack of orchitis
    REF: Ibid.

47. Undesired effects of testosterone therapy in adult males include
1. gynecomastia
2. stimulation of the growth of a preexisting prostatic carcinoma
3. cholestatic jaundice
4. bladder neck obstruction in older patients
REF: Ibid., p. 355

48. Complications of the long-term administration of estrogens include
1. increased tendency to develop venous thrombosis
2. increased tendency to develop carcinoma of the endometrium
3. decreased glucose tolerance
4. decreased bone mineralization
REF: Ibid., p. 414

49. Patients with Klinefelter's syndrome are
1. chromatin-negative on buccal smear
2. prone to develop gynecomastia
3. usually found to have testes of normal size
4. typically infertile with elevated levels of serum gonadotropins
REF: Ibid., pp. 335-336
Bondy, P.K. and Rosenberg, L.E. (Eds): *Duncan's Diseases of Metabolism, 8th Ed.,* W.B. Saunders Company, Philadelphia, 1979, p. 1567

98 / Endocrinology

Directions Summarized				
A	B	C	D	E
1, 2, 3 only	1, 3 only	2, 4 only	4 only	All are correct

50. The syndrome of hypogonadotropic hypogonadism
   1. is associated in men with a low plasma testosterone and low serum gonadotropins
   2. is associated with an increased incidence of anosmia or hyposmia
   3. is associated with a decreased rate of skeletal maturation and eunuchoid habitus when it occurs in childhood
   4. is associated with an increased incidence of gynecomastia

   REF: Williams, R.H. (Ed): *Textbook of Endocrinology, 5th Ed.,* W.B. Saunders Company, Philadelphia, 1974, p. 348
   Bondy, P.K. and Rosenberg, L.E. (Eds): *Duncan's Diseases of Metabolism, 8th Ed.,* W.B. Saunders Company, Philadelphia, 1979, p. 152

51. Testicular neoplasms
   1. are rarely malignant
   2. usually present as an enlargement of the testis
   3. are often associated with an increase in the urinary 17-ketosteroids
   4. are often associated with an increase in serum HCG or alpha-fetoprotein

   REF: Williams, R.H. (Ed): *Textbook of Endocrinology, 5th Ed.,* W.B. Saunders Company, Philadelphia, 1974, pp. 362-363
   Bondy, P.K. and Rosenberg, L.E. (Eds): *Duncan's Diseases of Metabolism, 8th Ed.,* W.B. Saunders Company, Philadelphia, 1979, p. 1575

52. In the polycystic ovary syndrome
1. plasma levels of testosterone and androstenedione are usually elevated
2. urinary 17-ketosteroids are usually within the normal range or borderline elevated
3. serum LH is often elevated
4. dexamethasone administration will suppress the urinary 17-ketosteroids, but often not as completely as in normal subjects
REF: Williams, R.H. (Ed): *Textbook of Endocrinology, 5th Ed.*, W.B. Saunders Company, Philadelphia, 1974, pp. 410-412

DIRECTIONS: Each of the questions or incomplete statements below is followed by five suggested answers or completions. Select the **one** that is **BEST** in each case.

V. Parathyroids and Bone Metabolism

53. The most common symptom in patients with primary hyperparathyroidism is
A. bone pain or fracture
B. hypertension
C. muscle weakness
D. passage of kidney stones
E. constipation
REF: Williams, R.H. (Ed): *Textbook of Endocrinology, 5th Ed.*, W.B. Saunders Company, Philadelphia, 1974, p. 736

DIRECTIONS: Each of the questions or incomplete statements below is followed by five suggested answers or completions. Select the **one** that is **BEST** in each case.

54. A 47-year-old woman complains of gradual weight loss with weakness and dull aching pain in the hips, back, and shoulders. Five years ago she underwent a subtotal gastrectomy for peptic ulcer disease. She now appears thin and chronically ill. There is diffuse tenderness to pressure exerted over the ribs or lumbar spine. Preliminary lab tests show a serum calcium of 6.8 mg/dl, phosphorus 2.0, BUN 12, albumin 2.8, total protein 5.8, alkaline phosphatase 15 units (normal less than 6 units) hematocrit 35%, white count 5,500. The most likely cause of her problem with calcium metabolism would be
    A. hypocalcemia accounted for by hypoproteinema due to poor nutrition
    B. multiple myeloma
    C. hypoparathyroidism
    D. renal osteodystrophy
    E. osteomalacia secondary to gastric surgery
    REF: Ibid., pp. 755-756
    Bondy, P.K. and Rosenberg, L.E. (Eds): *Duncan's Diseases of Metabolism, 8th Ed.,* W.B. Saunders Company, Philadelphia, 1979, pp. 1393-1394, 1400

55. The best choice of therapy for the patient in question 54 would be
   A. vitamin D, 10,000 units per week plus a calcium supplement
   B. vitamin D, 100,000 units per day plus a calcium supplement
   C. calcitonin, 50 units per day
   D. sodium phosphate, 1 g twice daily
   E. prednisone, 50 mg daily
   REF: Williams, R.H. (Ed): *Textbook of Endocrinology, 5th Ed.*, W.B. Saunders Company, Philadelphia, 1974, p. 756
   Bondy, P.K. and Rosenberg, L.E. (Eds): *Duncan's Diseases of Metabolism, 8th Ed.*, W.B. Saunders Company, Philadelphia, 1979, p. 1395

DIRECTIONS: For each of the following questions or incomplete statements, **ONE** or **MORE** of the answers or completions given is correct. Select:
- **A** if only 1, 2 and 3 are correct,
- **B** if only 1 and 3 are correct,
- **C** if only 2 and 4 are correct,
- **D** if only 4 is correct,
- **E** if all are correct.

56. The bone disease of primary hyperparathyroidism
    1. is most characteristically associated with subperiosteal bone resorption of the phalanges
    2. may be manifest only as a generalized loss of bone density on x-ray
    3. is associated with an increased rate of bone absorption
    4. can be distinguished microscopically from the bone disease associated with secondary hyperparathyroidism
    REF: Williams, R.H. (Ed): *Textbook of Endocrinology, 5th Ed.*, W.B. Saunders Company, Philadelphia, 1974, p. 737
    Bondy, P.K. and Rosenberg, L.E. (Eds): *Duncan's Diseases of Metabolism, 8th Ed.*, W.B. Saunders Company, Philadelphia, 1979, pp. 1344-1345

Endocrinology / 103

57. Secondary hyperparathyroidism
   1. is usually associated with elevated serum calcium levels
   2. is found in a variety of disease states where there is target-organ resistance to the action of parathyroid hormone (PTH)
   3. is characterized by autonomous secretion of PTH at greatly increased rates
   4. characteristically results in hyperplasia of all of the parathyroid gland
   REF: Williams, R.H. (Ed): *Textbook of Endocrinology, 5th Ed.*, W.B. Saunders Company, Philadelphia, 1974, pp. 754-759
   Bondy, P.K. and Rosenberg, L.E. (Eds): *Duncan's Diseases of Metabolism, 8th Ed.*, W.B. Saunders Company, Philadelphia, 1979, pp. 1363-1365

58. Pseudohypoparathyroidism differs from hypoparathyroidism in that
   1. parathyroid hormone levels in the blood are normal or elevated
   2. serum calcium and phosphorus are normal
   3. there is a subnormal rise in urinary cyclic AMP after the administration of PTH
   4. serum calcium can be normalized with physiologic replacement doses of vitamin D_2
   REF: Williams, R.H. (Ed): *Textbook of Endocrinology, 5th Ed.*, W.B. Saunders Company, Philadelphia, 1974, pp. 1341-1343

59. Osteoporosis is characterized by
   1. hypocalcemia
   2. hypophosphatemia
   3. elevated serum alkaline phosphatase
   4. generalized decrease in bone mass
   REF: Ibid., pp. 768-769
   Bondy, P.K. and Rosenberg, L.E. (Eds): *Duncan's Diseases of Metabolism, 8th Ed.*, W.B. Saunders Company, Philadelphia, 1979, pp. 1375-1377

	Directions Summarized			
A	B	C	D	E
1, 2, 3	1, 3	2, 4	4	All are
only	only	only	only	correct

60. Characteristic chemical findings in the blood of most patients with osteomalacia and normal kidneys include
   1. normal or low serum calcium
   2. elevated serum PTH
   3. elevated alkaline phosphatase
   4. normal serum phosphorus
   REF: Williams, R.H. (Ed): *Textbook of Endocrinology, 5th Ed.,* W.B. Saunders Company, Philadelphia, 1974, p. 756
   Bondy, P.K. and Rosenberg, L.E. (Eds): *Duncan's Diseases of Metabolism, 8th Ed.,* W.B. Saunders Company, Philadelphia, 1979, p. 1389

61. Laboratory tests that are consistently abnormal in Paget's disease of bone include
   1. serum calcium
   2. serum alkaline phosphatase
   3. renal phosphate clearance
   4. urinary hydroxyproline
   REF: Williams, R.H. (Ed): *Textbook of Endocrinology, 5th Ed.,* W.B. Saunders Company, Philadelphia, 1974, p. 767
   Bondy, P.K. and Rosenberg, L.E. (Eds): *Duncan's Diseases of Metabolism, 8th Ed.,* W.B. Saunders Company, Philadelphia, 1979, p. 1380

DIRECTIONS: Each of the questions or incomplete statements below is followed by five suggested answers or completions. Select the **one** that is **BEST** in each case.

VI. The Endocrine Pancreas, Diabetes, and Energy Metabolism

62. Which one of the findings below would provide the most conclusive evidence for the presence of an insulinoma?
    A. repeated fasting hypoglycemia
    B. repeated postprandial hypoglycemia
    C. pancreatic tumor demonstrated by angiography
    D. fasting blood glucose 45 mg/dl, serum immunoreactive insulin 30 μU/ml
    E. Blood glucose 45 mg/dl 30 minutes after intravenous tolbutamide, serum immunoreactive insulin 30 μU/ml
    REF: Williams, R.H. (Ed): *Textbook of Endocrinology, 5th Ed.,* W.B. Saunders Company, Philadelphia, 1974, p. 650

63. The ophthalmologic finding most suggestive of a high-risk of vitreous hemorrhage in the diabetic is
    A. microaneurysm
    B. waxy or hard exudate
    C. neovascularization
    D. cotton wool exudate
    E. lipemia retinalis
    REF: Ibid., p. 579
    Bondy, P.K. and Rosenberg, L.E. (Eds): *Duncan's Diseases of Metabolism, 8th Ed.,* W.B. Saunders Company, Philadelphia, 1979, p. 295

DIRECTIONS: For each of the following questions or incomplete statements, **ONE** or **MORE** of the answers or completions given is correct. Select:
    A if only 1, 2 and 3 are correct,
    B if only 1 and 3 are correct,
    C if only 2 and 4 are correct,
    D if only 4 is correct,
    E if all are correct.

64. In contrast to the normal β cell, the insulinoma
 1. shows a relatively greater stimulation by glucagon than by glucose
 2. shows a relatively greater stimulation by tolbutamide than by glucose
 3. continues to secret insulin inappropriately at very low blood glucose concentrations
 4. may secrete a relatively large proportion of hormone as proinsulin

 REF: Williams, R.H. (Ed): *Textbook of Endocrinology, 5th Ed.,* W.B. Saunders Company, Philadelphia, 1974, p. 650
       Marble, A., et al. (Eds): *Joslin's Diabetes Mellitus, 11th Ed.,* Lea & Febiger, Philadelphia, 1971, p. 800

Endocrinology / 107

65. True glycosuria (as detected by the glucose oxidase method)
1. may be seen in nondiabetic individuals who have normal levels of blood glucose
2. is always seen in diabetic individuals when their blood glucose levels are elevated
3. occurs in most subjects when blood glucose levels exceed 180-200 mg/dl
4. is found in two uncommon hereditary disorders, essential pentosuria and essential fructosuria

REF: Williams, R.H. (Ed): *Textbook of Endocrinology, 5th Ed.,* W.B. Saunders Company, Philadelphia, 1974, p. 560
Bondy, P.K. and Rosenberg, L.E. (Eds): *Duncan's Diseases of Metabolism, 8th Ed.,* W.B. Saunders Company, Philadelphia, 1979, p. 252

66. Obesity is a contributory factor in the development of diabetes because
1. it decreases the early phase of insulin secretion after glucose
2. it is associated with an increased rate of insulin degradation
3. it is usually associated with a supranormal dietary intake of carbohydrates
4. peripheral tissues are less responsive to insulin in the presence of obesity

REF: Ibid., p. 248
Stanbury, J.B., Wyngaarden, J.B., Frederickson, D.S. (Eds): *The Metabolic Basis of Inherited Disease, 4th Ed.,* McGraw-Hill Book Company, New York, 1978, pp. 86-89

Directions Summarized				
A	B	C	D	E
1, 2, 3 only	1, 3 only	2, 4 only	4 only	All are correct

67. Increasing requirements for insulin in a diabetic may be a result of
    1. infection
    2. glucocorticoid therapy
    3. high titers of insulin antibodies
    4. repeated episodes of hypoglycemia
    REF: Bondy, P.K. and Rosenberg, L.E. (Eds): *Duncan's Diseases of Metabolism, 8th Ed.,* W.B. Saunders Company, Philadelphia, 1979, p. 276
    Williams, R.H. (Ed): *Textbook of Endocrinology, 5th Ed.,* W.B. Saunders Company, Philadelphia, 1974, pp. 592-593

68. Pregnancy in a diabetic woman
    1. will tend to cause increased resistance to insulin
    2. will tend to lower the renal threshold for glucose, causing increased glycosuria
    3. will tend to cause more rapid lipolysis and gluconeogenesis during short periods of fasting
    4. is associated with the rapid advancement of diabetic retinopathy and nephropathy in most patients
    REF: Bondy, P.K. and Rosenberg, L.E. (Eds): *Duncan's Diseases of Metabolism, 8th Ed.,* W.B. Saunders Company, Philadelphia, 1979, pp. 302-303
    Williams, R.H. (Ed): *Textbook of Endocrinology, 5th Ed.,* W.B. Saunders Company, Philadelphia, 1974, pp. 587-588

69. In uncontrolled diabetes the polyol or sorbitol pathway
1. becomes more active as a pathway of glucose metabolism
2. leads to intracellular accumulation of osmotically active substances that cannot diffuse freely from cells
3. probably accounts for the fluctuations in visual acuity seen with marked hyperglycemia
4. may account for the occurrence of cerebral edema occasionally seen during the treatment of diabetic ketoacidosis

REF: Bondy, P.K. and Rosenberg, L.E. (Eds): *Duncan's Diseases of Metabolism, 8th Ed.,* W.B. Saunders Company, Philadelphia, 1979, pp. 290-291
Williams, R.H. (Ed): *Textbook of Endocrinology, 5th Ed.,* W.B. Saunders Company, Philadelphia, 1974, p. 606
Stanbury, J.B., Wyngaarden, J.B., Frederickson, D.S. (Eds): *The Metabolic Basis of Inherited Disease, 4th Ed.,* McGraw-Hill Book Company, New York, 1978, p. 102

70. Untreated diabetic acidosis is commonly associated with
1. marked resistance to the peripheral effects of insulin, so that over 200 units per day are required
2. immunoreactive insulin levels less than 5 μU/ml
3. hyperchloremia
4. hyperventilation

REF: Bondy, P.K. and Rosenberg, L.E. (Eds): *Duncan's Diseases of Metabolism, 8th Ed.,* W.B. Saunders Company, Philadelphia, 1979, p. 285
Marble, A., et al. (Eds): *Joslin's Diabetes Mellitus, 11th Ed.,* Lea & Febiger, Philadelphia, 1971, pp. 370-371, 374-375

110 / Endocrinology

	Directions Summarized			
A	B	C	D	E
1, 2, 3 only	1, 3 only	2, 4 only	4 only	All are correct

71. In comparison to ketoacidotic coma, hyperosmolar diabetic coma is associated
    1. with the maintenance of a greater capability for insulin secretion
    2. more frequently with seizures
    3. with higher elevations of blood glucose
    4. with higher rates of lipolysis
    REF: Bondy, P.K. and Rosenberg, L.E. (Eds): *Duncan's Diseases of Metabolism, 8th Ed.,* W.B. Saunders Company, Philadelphia, 1979, p. 292
    Williams, R.H. (Ed): *Textbook of Endocrinology, 5th Ed.,* W.B. Saunders Company, Philadelphia, 1974, p. 609

72. The infusion of sodium bicarbonate in a patient with diabetic ketoacidosis
    1. is usually required, since insulin therapy alone cannot correct the acidosis
    2. is preferable to sodium lactate infusion for the amelioration of severe acidosis
    3. will cause a prompt rise in the pH of both the arterial blood and the cerebrospinal fluid
    4. will cause a prompt rise in the pH of the arterial blood, but a fall in the pH of the cerebrospinal fluid
    REF: Bondy, P.K. and Rosenberg, L.E. (Eds): *Duncan's Diseases of Metabolism, 8th Ed.,* W.B. Saunders Company, Philadelphia, 1979, pp. 289-291

73. A patient presents with blood glucose 200 mg/dl, ketones positive only in undiluted serum, serum CO_2 8 mM, and arterial pH 7.2. These data are compatible with
   1. acute diabetic ketoacidosis
   2. alcohol ingestion in a patient with mild diabetes
   3. starvation ketosis
   4. lactic acidosis in a patient with mild diabetes
   REF: Ibid., pp. 1542-1545
   Marble, A., et al. (Eds): *Joslin's Diabetes Mellitus, 11th Ed.,* Lea & Febiger, Philadelphia, 1971, p. 390

74. Renal failure in the diabetic is
   1. more commonly the cause of death in juvenile-onset than in maturity-onset diabetes
   2. most often a result of diabetic glomerulosclerosis
   3. unlikely to be caused by glomerulosclerosis in the absence of demonstrable retinopathy
   4. frequently exacerbated by urinary infection
   REF: Ibid., pp. 536-540

75. A 30-year-old diabetic man takes 40 units of NPH insulin each morning and follows a regular 2,400 calorie diet. His weight is normal, and he has no long-term diabetic complications. Tests for urine glucose are consistently 3 to 4+ before breakfast but are negative before lunch and supper. He has mild hypoglycemic symptoms in the late afternoon three or four times per week. Which of the following would represent reasonable alterations in his diabetic management?
   1. reduce the caloric intake to 2,000 calories per day
   2. increase the morning dose of NPH to 45 units
   3. add 5 units of regular insulin to the morning dose
   4. reduce the morning dose of insulin by 3 units and add 6 units of NPH insulin at supper time
   REF: Williams, R.H. (Ed): *Textbook of Endocrinology, 5th Ed.,* W.B. Saunders Company, Philadelphia, 1974, p. 591

VI: Rheumatology

DIRECTIONS: Each of the questions or incomplete statements below is followed by five suggested answers or completions. Select the **one** that is **BEST** in each case.

1. The most frequent cause of fungal arthritis is
   A. coccidioidomycosis
   B. histoplasmosis
   C. blastomycosis
   D. cryptococcosis
   E. sporotrichosis
   REF: Supplement to the Journal of the American Medical Association 224:5:661–812, April 30, 1973, p. 755

2. All the following are true of Caffey's disease (infantile cortical hyperostosis) EXCEPT
   A. the mandible is most frequently affected
   B. normal serum alkaline phosphatase activity is a characteristic
   C. there is an increase in the size of the bone, prinicipally in the diaphysis
   D. steroids have a profound effect
   E. the disease is usually self-limited
   REF: Ibid., pp. 780-781

3. All the following diseases are characterized as intermittent arthritis syndromes EXCEPT
   A. systemic lupus erythematosus
   B. gout
   C. palindromic rheumatism
   D. familial Mediterranean fever
   E. Whipple's disease
   REF: Moscowitz, R.W.: *Clinical Rheumatology: A Problem-Oriented Approach to Diagnosis and Management*, Lea & Febiger, Philadelphia, 1975, p. 116

4. The inflammatory arteritides include all the following EXCEPT
   A. polyarteritis nodosa
   B. hypersensitivity angiitis
   C. rheumatic fever arteritis
   D. allergic granulomatous arteritis
   E. thrombotic thrombocytopenia purpura
   REF: Dick, W.C.: *An Introduction to Clinical Rheumatology,* Williams and Williams, Baltimore, 1972, p. 93

5. In a previously unsensitized person, how many days after injection of a foreign serum can the most common reaction be expected to occur?
   A. 1-2
   B. 3-5
   C. 6
   D. 7-12
   E. 14 or more
   REF: Supplement to the Journal of the American Medical Association 224:5:661-812, April 30, 1973, p. 726

6. Polymyalgia rheumatica
   A. is more common in women than men
   B. is associated with hypochromic anemia
   C. is characterized by a normal erythrocyte sedimentation rate
   D. evolves to temporal arteritis in less than 10% of cases
   E. has few constitutional symptoms
   REF: Dick, W.C.: *An Introduction to Clinical Rheumatology,* Williams and Wilkins, Baltimore, 1972, p. 159

7. All the following are true of de Quervain's tenosynovitis EXCEPT
   A. it is a tenosynovitis of the abductor pollicis longus and extensor brevis pollicis at the wrist
   B. in most patients this disorder is primary and related to chronic nonspecific trauma
   C. maximal pain is induced by forced radial deviation after the thumb has been placed in the palm of the hand and grasped by the fingers
   D. the patient complains of pain with use of the thumb or wrist
   E. physical examination reveals severe tenderness and occasionally signs of inflammation over the tendon
   REF: Moscowitz, R.W.: *Clinical Rheumatology: A Problem-Oriented Approach to Diagnosis and Management,* Lea & Febiger, Philadelphia, 1975, p. 202

8. The most clinical feature of Reiter's syndrome is
   A. urethritis
   B. conjunctivitis
   C. arthritis
   D. prostatitis
   E. sacroiliitis
   REF: Dick, W.C.: *An Introduction to Clinical Rheumatology*, Williams and Wilkins, Baltimore, 1972, p. 114

9. All the following are characteristic of Whipple's disease EXCEPT
   A. fever
   B. abdominal pain
   C. constipation
   D. cutaneous hyperpigmentation
   E. adenopathy
   REF: Moscowitz, R.W.: *Clinical Rheumatology: A Problem-Oriented Approach to Diagnosis and Management*, Lea & Febiger, Philadelphia, 1975, p. 118

10. All of the following are commonly affected by the degenerative process of osteoarthrosis EXCEPT
    A. the distal interphalangeal joints of the fingers
    B. the first metacarpophalangeal and carpometacarpal joints of the thumb
    C. the upper part of the cervical spine
    D. the lumbosacral spine
    E. the large weight-bearing regions (hips, knees, and first metatarsophalangeal joints)
    REF: Postgrad. Med. 65:64–66, 1979

11. All the following are true of rheumatoid factor (RF) EXCEPT
    A. it is an IgM globulin that has the capacity to react with IgG globulins *in vitro*
    B. there are other antiglobulins of the IgG and IgA variety
    C. the stimulus for the production of RF is not known
    D. it is found in the sera and synovial fluid of adult patients with established rheumatoid arthritis
    E. it is usually seen in juvenile rheumatoid arthritis
    REF: Bellanti, J.A.: *Immunology II*, W.B. Saunders Company, Philadelphia, 1978, pp. 575–576

12. Soft-tissue rheumatism syndromes
    A. are rare
    B. are commonly indicative of generalized disease
    C. are characterized by generalized areas of musculoskeletal pain and tenderness
    D. include such syndromes as tennis elbow, supraspinatous capsulitis, and trochanteric bursitis
    E. radiographs usually reveal extensive soft-tissue calcification
    REF: Postgrad. Med. 65:64–66, 1979

13. Drugs that raise serum uric acid include
    A. probenecid
    B. coumarin derivatives
    C. phenylbutazone
    D. adrenal corticosteroids
    E. none of the above
    REF: Moskowitz, R.W.: *Clinical Rheumatology: A Problem-Oriented Approach to Diagnosis and Management*, Lea & Febiger, Philadelphia, 1975, p. 24

14. In patients with pseudogout which of the following are most frequently involved?
   A. wrists
   B. shoulders
   C. ankles
   D. elbows
   E. knees
   REF: Ibid., p. 57

15. All the following occur in association with the Lesch-Nyhan syndrome EXCEPT
   A. choreoathetosis
   B. spasticity
   C. mental retardation
   D. self-mutilation
   E. overproduction of HG-PRTase
   REF: Supplement to the Journal of the American Medical Association 224:5:661–812, April 30, 1973, p. 761

16. In polymyalgia rheumatica
   A. younger age groups are affected
   B. pain and stiffness occur mainly in distal muscles
   C. morning stiffness is marked
   D. muscle atrophy is common
   E. alpha-2 globulin and fibrinogen are usually decreased
   REF: Ibid., p. 728

17. All the following are true of intermittent hydrarthrosis EXCEPT
    A. although attacks are usually monoarticular, polyarticular involvement does occur
    B. the interval between attacks varies from one week to one month, with intervals of one to two weeks being most common
    C. attacks at monthly intervals are likely to be related to menstruation in women
    D. laboratory findings confirm the diagnosis
    E. in some patients, effusions cease after many years; other patients will have the syndrome as a lifelong condition
    REF: Moskowitz, R.W.: *Clinical Rheumatology: A Problem-Oriented Approach to Diagnosis and Management*, Lea & Febiger, Philadelphia, 1975, p. 118

18. Which of the following in association with pneumoconiosis may give a picture of multiple, well-defined, hard round shadows scattered throughout both lung fields (Caplan's syndrome)?
    A. progressive systemic sclerosis
    B. systemic lupus erythematosus
    C. polyarteritis nodosa
    D. rheumatoid arthritis
    E. none of the above
    REF: Boyle, A.C.: *Color Atlas of Rheumatology*, Year Book Medical Publishers, Inc., Chicago, 1974, p. 38

19. Noncartilaginous manifestations of relapsing polychondritis include all the following EXCEPT
    A. fever
    B. iritis, episcleritis, and cataracts
    C. deafness
    D. aortic stenosis
    E. anemia
    REF: Supplement to the Journal of the American Medical Association 224:5:661-812, April 30, 1973, p. 728

120 / Rheumatology

20. All the following are true of osteoarthritis EXCEPT
    A. the major lesion in affected joints is in articular cartilage, which shows softening, fibrillation, and flaking
    B. the underlying causes of joint changes are obscure, but it appears that both mechanical and biochemical factors play a part
    C. subchondral bone undergoes thickening and sclerosis, and cysts may occur in deeper layers, perhaps owing to herniation of synovial fluid through breaks in the trabeculae
    D. osteophyte formation at the margin of affected joints is characteristic
    E. there are signs of inflammation in affected joints
    REF: Boyle, A.C.: *Color Atlas of Rheumatology*, Year Book Medical Publishers, Inc., Chicago, 1974, p. 75

21. Evidence of sarcoid includes all the following EXCEPT
    A. positive tuberculin skin test
    B. hilar adenopathy
    C. iritis and parotid swelling
    D. fever
    E. skin rash
    REF: Moskowitz, R.W.: *Clinical Rheumatology: A Problem-Oriented Approach to Diagnosis and Management*, Lea & Febiger, Philadelphia, 1975, p. 88

22. The most serious complication of systemic lupus erythematosus is
    A. arthritis
    B. pleuritis
    C. peritonitis
    D. renal involvement
    E. pericarditis
    REF: Boyle, A.C.: *Color Atlas of Rheumatology*, Year Book Medical Publishers, Inc., Chicago, 1974, p. 96

23. All the following are main features of ankylosing spondylitis EXCEPT
    A. a marked female predominance with onset in the late teens or early twenties
    B. bilateral sacroiliitis usually proceeding to paraspinal ligamentous calcification or ossification with ankylosis of the spinal facet joints
    C. peripheral joint involvement more common in the hips and shoulders than elsewhere
    D. a high incidence (about 25%) of iritis
    E. rarely, aortitis or pulmonary fibrosis affecting the upper lung fields may occur
    REF: Ibid., p. 51

24. In what percent of patients with complete agammaglobulinemia does a rheumatoid arthritis-like disease develop, usually in the absence of serum rheumatoid factor?
    A. 10%
    B. 30%
    C. 50%
    D. 70%
    E. 90%
    REF: Postgrad. Med. 65:64–80, 1979

25. All the following are true of intermittent hydrarthrosis EXCEPT
    A. it is characterized by acute recurrent attacks of joint swelling of predictable periodicity
    B. joint effusions are notable for their lack of local inflammatory change and relatively little pain
    C. systemic signs and symptoms are present
    D. usually, symptoms completely resolve, and attacks abate in two to four days
    E. knees are involved most commonly
    REF: Moskowitz, R.W.: *Clinical Rheumatology: A Problem-Oriented Approach to Diagnosis and Management*, Lea & Febiger, Philadelphia, 1975, p. 118

26. In ankylosing spondylitis
    A. hypochromic anemia is present in most cases
    B. rheumatoid factor is frequently present
    C. the earliest x-ray changes are seen in the sacroiliac joints
    D. the sacroiliac joints rarely become fused
    E. none of the above
    REF: Supplement to the Journal of the American Medical Association 224:5:661-812, April 30, 1973, p. 730

27. Side effects of steroids include all the following EXCEPT
    A. hyperkalemia
    B. cataracts, glaucoma
    C. fat redistribution
    D. myopathy
    E. peptic ulcer complications
    REF: Dick, W.C.: *An Introduction to Clinical Rheumatology*, Williams and Wilkins, Baltimore, 1972, p. 177

28. All the following are true of palindromic rheumatism EXCEPT
    A. it is characterized by acute, abrupt attacks of joint inflammation
    B. symptoms often develop within a period of hours
    C. severe pain occurs early, followed by joint redness, tenderness, and swelling
    D. any peripheral joint may be affected
    E. joint pain increases when swelling is maximal
    REF: Moskowitz, R.W.: *Clinical Rheumatology: A Problem-Oriented Approach to Diagnosis and Management*, Lea & Febiger, Philadelphia, 1975, p. 117

29. All the following are characteristic of osteogenesis imperfecta EXCEPT
   A. it is an autosomal dominant trait
   B. osteoporosis and fractures
   C. blue sclerae
   D. ligamentous laxity
   E. thick skin
   REF: Dick, W.C.: *An Introduction to Clinical Rheumatology*, Williams and Wilkins, Baltimore, 1972, p. 166

DIRECTIONS: For each of the following questions or incomplete statements, ONE or MORE of the answers or completions given is correct. Select:
   A if only 1, 2 and 3 are correct,
   B if only 1 and 3 are correct,
   C if only 2 and 4 are correct,
   D if only 4 is correct,
   E if all are correct.

30. In rheumatoid arthritis
   1. mononeuritis multiplex may occur as a result of necrotizing arteritis affecting the vasa nervorum
   2. if pericarditis develops it is usually symptomatic
   3. hemoglobin and plasma iron levels tend to revert toward normal as disease activity lessens
   4. conservative measures are unwarranted at the outset of treatment
   REF: Supplement to the Journal of the American Medical Association 224:5:661-812, April 30, 1973, pp. 694-696

Directions Summarized				
A	B	C	D	E
1, 2, 3 only	1, 3 only	2, 4 only	4 only	All are correct

31. Concerning McArdle's disease
    1. it is a hereditary disorder characterized by an excess of muscle phosphorylase
    2. it is associated with muscle weakness and pain due to inability of muscle to metabolize glycogen for energy
    3. samples of venous blood drawn from the arm during muscle use usually reveal an increased production of lactic acid as an end-product of glycogen metabolism
    4. myoglobinuria is common
    REF: Moskowitz, R.W.: *Clinical Rheumatology: A Problem-Oriented Approach to Diagnosis and Management*, Lea & Febiger, Philadelphia, 1975, pp. 131–132

32. Factors associated with a poor prognosis in rheumatoid arthritis with respect to joint function include
    1. persistent disease of more than one year's duration
    2. high titers of rheumatoid factor
    3. presence of subcutaneous nodules
    4. age above 30 when the patient is first seen by a physician
    REF: Supplement to the Journal of the American Medical Association 224:5:661–812, April 30, 1973, p. 695

33. Osteoarthritis
    1. is unrelated to occupation
    2. is about equally common in women and men
    3. is associated with an elevated erythrocyte sedimentation rate
    4. as a severe disease, is more common in women
    REF: Dick, W.C.: *An Introduction to Clinical Rheumatology*, Williams and Wilkins, Baltimore, 1972, pp. 12–13

34. Regarding acute monoarthritis due to trauma or internal derangement
    1. joint rest is important in the management
    2. elastic compression bandages are helpful
    3. surgical intervention may be indicated if ligament or cartilage injury is present
    4. cold applications are not advisable, especially in the early stages
    REF: Moskowitz, R.W.: *Clinical Rheumatology: A Problem-Oriented Approach to Diagnosis and Management*, Lea & Febiger, Philadelphia, 1975, p. 63

35. The typical pattern of distribution for ankylosing spondylitis includes the
    1. sacroiliac joints
    2. intervertebral disk spaces
    3. apophyseal and costovertebral joints
    4. symphysis pubis
    REF: Postgrad. Med. 65:64–69, 1979

36. Tests that measure the number and function of T cells include
    1. absolute lymphocyte count
    2. rosette formation with sheep erythrocytes (E rosettes)
    3. development of delayed hypersensitivity to mumps, *Candida, Trichophyton*, purified protein derivative of tuberculin, streptokinase-streptodornase
    4. development of contact allergy to dinitrochlorobenzene
    REF: American College of Physicians: *Medical Knowldege Self-Assessment: Program IV: Syllabus, 1977: Recent Developments in Internal Medicine*, American College of Physicians, Philadelphia, 1976, p. 264

Directions Summarized				
A	B	C	D	E
1, 2, 3 only	1, 3 only	2, 4 only	4 only	All are correct

37. In akylosing spolitis
    1. no obvious relationship is found between activity of spondylitis and iritis
    2. the most common cardiac conduction disturbance is complete atrioventricular block
    3. the incidence of aortic insufficiency is correlated with extent and duration of joint involvement
    4. aortic insufficiency develops in over 10% of cases
    REF: Supplement to the Journal of the American Medical Association 224:5:661–812, April 30, 1973, p. 730

38. Organized dense fibrous tissue includes
    1. tendons
    2. aponeuroses
    3. ligaments
    4. periosteum
    REF: Ibid., p. 670

39. In sickle cell disease
    1. crises are rarely associated with polyarthralgia
    2. patients are increasingly susceptible to *Salmonella* osteomyelitis
    3. hydrarthroses do not occur
    4. hyperuricemia and secondary gouty arteritis may occur
    REF: Supplement to the Journal of the American Medical Association 224:5:661–812, April 30, 1973, p. 772

40. Concerning Paget's disease
1. destruction and remodeling leads to enlargement and softening of bone
2. affects 1%-3% of persons past age 45
3. pelvis, femur, skull, tibia and vertebrae are most commonly affected
4. most often monostatic
REF: Ibid., p. 103

41. Which of the following is true of pachydermoperiostosis?
1. young males are primarily affected
2. joints are swollen and tender
3. it is characterized by thick dense periostosis
4. it is related to underlying disease
REF: Dick, W.C.: *An Introduction to Clinical Rheumatology*, Williams and Wilkins, Baltimore, 1972, p. 153

42. Avascular necrosis of the head of the femur may occur in individuals with
1. sickle cell trait
2. sickle cell C disease
3. sickle cell thalassemia
4. sickle cell S disease
REF: Supplement to the Journal of the American Medical Association 224:5:661-812, April 30, 1973, p. 772

43. Which of the following is (are) true of rheumatic fever?
1. with most attacks, signs of acute inflammation subside within six weeks
2. valvular lesions may heal completely
3. complete subsidence of arthritis without residual joint abnormality is the rule
4. within the first two months of the attack, less than 50% of patients have an increased antistreptolysin O titer
REF: Ibid., pp. 737-738

	Directions Summarized			
A	B	C	D	E
1, 2, 3 only	1, 3 only	2, 4 only	4 only	All are correct

44. Regarding the scalenus anticus syndrome
    1. pressure on the neurovascular bundle may be caused by compression of the bundle between the scalenus anticus muscle and a normal first rib
    2. hypertrophy and spastic irritability of the muscle are often present
    3. paresthesia and vasomotor disturbances such as Raynaud's phenomena are common
    4. pain extends from the neck to the hand, usually in a radial distribution
    REF: Moskowitz, R.W.: *Clinical Rheumatology: A Problem-Oriented Approach to Diagnosis and Management*, Lea & Febiger, Philadelphia, 1975, p. 207

45. Common manifestations of Behcet's disease include
    1. recurrent painful orogenital ulcers and eye inflammation
    2. arthritis
    3. thrombophlebitis
    4. neurologic abnormalities
    REF: American College of Physicians: *Medical Knowledge Self-Assessment: Program IV: Syllabus, 1977: Recent Developments in Internal Medicine*, American College of Physicians, Philadelphia, 1976, p. 277

46. Peak onset of dermatomyositis occurs in
    1. childhood
    2. the second to fourth decade
    3. the fourth to sixth decade
    4. the sixth to eighth decade
    REF: Dick. W.C.: *An Introduction to Clinical Rheumatology*, Williams and Wilkins, Baltimore, 1972, p. 86

47. Patients with "secondary" amyloid often have deposits in
    1. kidneys
    2. spleen
    3. liver
    4. adrenals
    REF: American College of Physicians: *Medical Knowledge Self-Assessment: Program IV: Syllabus, 1977: Recent Developments in Internal Medicine*, American College of Physicians, Philadelphia, 1976, p. 273

48. The anti-inflammatory effects of steroids include
    1. increased antibody formation
    2. impaired cell-mediated immunity
    3. increased circulating eosinophils
    4. reduction of lymphoid tissue
    REF: Dick, W.C.: *An Introduction to Clinical Rheumatology*, Williams and Wilkins, Baltimore, 1972, p. 177

49. Abnormal findings on urinalysis favor a diagnosis of
    1. systemic lupus erythematosus
    2. vasculitis
    3. scleroderma
    4. rheumatoid arthritis
    REF: Moskowitz, R.W.: *Clinical Rheumatology: A Problem-Oriented Approach to Diagnosis and Management*, Lea & Febiger, Philadelphia, 1975, p. 22

50. Patients with gout should be instructed to
    1. decrease fluid intake
    2. lose weight rapidly
    3. take at least four aspirin per day
    4. avoid alcohol excess
    REF: Dick, W.C.: *An Introduction to Clinical Rheumatology*, Williams and Wilkins, Baltimore, 1972, p. 129

VII: Nephrology

DIRECTIONS: Each of the questions or incomplete statements below is followed by suggested answers or completions. Select the **BEST** answer(s) in each case.

1. Which one of the following statements about alcoholic ketoacidosis is FALSE?
   A. the NADH/NAD ratio is increased
   B. the acetoacetate/β-hydroxybutyrate ratio is decreased
   C. glucose is the most effective treatment, and addition of either insulin or bicarbonate is usually unnecessary
   D. hyperphosphatemia is common on admission
   E. alcohol levels are usually normal on admission
   REF: Schrier, R.W. (Ed.): *Renal and Electrolyte Disorders,* Little, Brown and Company, Boston, 1976, p. 95

2. The descending limb of Henle is most permeable to
   A. sodium
   B. chloride
   C. urea
   D. water
   E. bicarbonate
   REF: Brenner, B.H. and Rector, F.C. (Eds.): *The Kidney,* W.B. Saunders Company, Philadelphia, 1976, p. 284

3. Diabetes insipidus, rather than compulsive polydipsia, is more likely if
   A. plasma osmolality is 260 mOsm/kg water
   B. the patient is a woman with a history of psychiatric disorder
   C. there is considerable variation in water intake
   D. the onset of the disorder is sudden
   E. the polyuria responds to fluid restriction
   REF: Schrier, R.W. (Ed.): *Renal and Electrolyte Disorders,* Little, Brown and Company, Boston, 1976, p. 15

4. Which of the following antidiuretic drugs may act directly on the kidney?
   A. clofibrate
   B. nicotine
   C. morphine
   D. chlorpropamide
   E. carbamazepine
   REF: Brenner, B.M. and Stein, J.H. (Eds.):1. *Sodium and Water Homeostasis,* 2. *Acid-Base and Potassium Homeostasis,* Churchill Livingstone, New York 1978, p. 12

5. A patient has a serum sodium of 170 mEq/l and a urine sodium of 10 mEq/l. The most likely cause is
   A. infusion of hypertonic saline
   B. water deprivation
   C. tube feeding
   D. diabetes insipidus
   E. diuretic abuse
   REF: Maxwell, M.H. and Kleeman, C.R.: *Clinical Disorders of Fluid and Electrolyte Metabolism, 2nd Ed.,* McGraw-Hill Book Company, New York, 1972, p. 99

6. If a patient with acidosis has a pH of 7.2 and a HCO_3^- of 10, how much bicarbonate will be required to raise his serum bicarbonate to 18, if his body weight is 60 kg?
   A. 8 mEq
   B. 680 mEq
   C. 48 mEq
   D. 240 mEq
   E. 27 mEq
   REF: Rose, B.H.: *Clincial Physiology of Acid-Base and Electrolyte Disorders,* McGraw-Hill Book Company, New York, 1977, p. 343

7. In a pure metabolic acidosis, if the plasma HCO_3^- is 14, the PCO_2 should be
   A. 52 mm
   B. 40 mm
   C. 28 mm
   D. 10 mm
   E. 18 mm
   REF: Ibid., p. 325

8. A patient with chronic metabolic acidosis receiving alkali therapy may hyperventilate for several days after the acidosis is corrected. Which one of the following findings would be most consistent with such a state?
   A. pH 7.4, PCO_2 40, HCO_3^- 24
   B. pH 7.5, PCO_2 40, HCO_3^- 30
   C. pH 7.5, PCO_2 20, HCO_3^- 16
   D. pH 7.3, PCO_2 30, HCO_3^- 14
   E. pH 7.5, PCO_2 50, HCO_3^- 36
   REF: Maxwell, M.H. and Kleeman, C.R.: *Clinical Disorders of Fluid and Electrolyte Metabolism, 2nd Ed.,* McGraw-Hill Book Company, New York, 1972, p. 321

9. With respect to urate, large doses of salicylates in man cause
A. suppression of secretion only
B. suppression of reabsorption only
C. suppression of secretion and reabsorption
D. increases reabsorption and suppresses secretion
E. suppresses reabsorption and increases secretion
REF: Pitts, R.F.: *Physiology of the Kidney and Body Fluids, 3rd Ed.*, Year Book Medical Publishers, Chicago, 1974, p. 88

10. Which of the following physiologic effects suggest a proximal tubular site of action for a diuretic?
A. significant phosphaturia
B. depression of free water clearance
C. hyperkalemia
D. a fractional bicarbonate excretion greater than 0.2
E. metabolic alkalosis
REF: Berliner, R.W. and Orloff, J. (Eds.): *Handbook of Physiology, Section 8-Renal Physiology,* Williams and Wilkins, Baltimore, 1973, p. 1005

11. Chronic thiazide administration may cause all of the following EXCEPT
A. hypomagnesuria
B. hypocalcuria
C. hypouricuria
D. hypokalemia
E. alkalosis
REF: Hamburger, J. et al. (Eds.): *Advances in Nephrology, Vol. 104*, Year Book Medical Publishers, Chicago, 1971-74
Beeson, P.B. McDermott, W., Wyngaarden, J.B. (Eds.): *Cecil Textbook of Medicine, 15th Ed.*, W.B. Saunders Company, Philadelphia, 1979

12. Full natriuretic action of spironolactone is evident within
    A. 10 to 30 minutes
    B. 2 to 4 hours
    C. 12 to 20 hours
    D. a few days
    E. none of the above
    REF: Black, D. (Ed.): *Renal Disease, 3rd Ed.*, Blackwell Scientific Publications, Oxford, London, 1972, p. 679

13. Urine specific gravity is LEAST influenced by
    A. glucose
    B. dextran
    C. protein
    D. pyelography dye
    REF: Papper, S.: *Clinical Nephrology, 2nd Ed.*, Little, Brown and Company, Boston, 1978, p. 7

14. An increase of the urinary specific gravity out of proportion to the expected osmolality would NOT occur in which one of the following?
    A. severe proteinuria
    B. contrast media from pyelography
    C. detergents used to clear the hydrometer
    D. testing urine at body temperature
    E. glycosuria
    REF: DeWardner, H.E.: *The Kidney: An Outline of Normal and Abnormal Structure and Function, 4th Ed.*, Longman, Inc., New York, 1973, p. 55

15. A low complement is seen in all of the following EXCEPT
    A. membranous glomerulonephritis
    B. mesangiocapillary glomerulonephritis
    C. bacterial endocarditis
    D. shunt nephritis
    E. systemic lupus erythematosus
    REF: Jenis, E.H. and Lowenthal, D.T.: *Kidney Biopsy Interpretation*, F.A. Davis Company, Philadelphia, 1977, p. 35

16. A 45-year-old diabetic has been treated for several years with tolbutamide. He has no retinopathy, and an intravenous pyelogram done ten days earlier was normal. A random urinalysis using Albustix is normal, but a plus 2 reaction is obtained with sulfosalicylic acid. The most likely explanation for the findings is
   A. diabetic nephropathy
   B. a false positive reaction to IVP dye
   C. a false positive reaction to tolbutamide
   D. mild renal damage from the IVP
   E. tubular proteinuria
   REF: Eurley, L.E. and Gottschalk, C.W.: *Strauss and Welts' Disease of the Kidney, 3rd Ed.*, Little, Brown and Company, Boston, 1979, p. 767

17. The next most useful step would be
   A. repeat the pyelogram
   B. examine an overnight specimen
   C. measure the 24-hour urine protein excretion
   D. measure creatinine clearance
   E. perform a renal biopsy
   REF: Ibid.

18. The 24-hour urinary protein excretion is 2.5 g. The next step would be which of the following?
   A. stop the tolbutamide
   B. bone marrow biopsy
   C. liver biopsy
   D. kidney biopsy
   E. measure protein selectivity
   REF: Ibid.

19. Atheromatous stenosis of the renal artery
   A. diffusely involves the renal artery
   B. appears as a "string of beads"
   C. usually involves the proximal ⅓ of the renal artery
   D. is rarely bilateral
   E. does not have poststenotic dilatation
   REF: Genest, J.: *Hypertension*, McGraw-Hill Book Company, New York, 1977, p. 820

20. The renin system is probably important in all of the following types of hypertension EXCEPT
   A. renovascular hypertension
   B. malignant hypertension
   C. renal infarction
   D. "page" kidney
   E. licorice-induced hypertension
   REF: Ibid., p. 559

21. In a patient who is hypokalemic off diuretics, which one of the following results would make primary aldosteronism likely?
   A. urine sodium 120 mEq/24 hr and urine potassium 12 mEq/24 hr
   B. urine sodium 200 mEq/24 hr and urine potassium 20 mEq/24 hr
   C. urine sodium 120 mEq/24 hr and urine potassium 20 mEq/24 hr
   D. urine sodium 80 mEq/24 hr and urine potassium 40 mEq/24 hr
   E. urine sodium 50 mEq/24 hr and urine potassium 20 mEq/24 hr
   REF: Ibid., p. 437

22. Administration of Sar[1] Ala[8] angiotensin II to a hypertensive patient results in an initial increase of blood pressure followed by a rapid decline both before and after salt depletion. This hypertension is most likely
   A. neurogenic in origin
   B. volume dependent
   C. associated with high plasma renin
   D. labile
   E. factions
   REF: Ibid., p. 187

23. A patient is found to have a blood pressure measurement by cuff of 160/70. His mean arterial pressure is approximately
   A. 120 mm
   B. 100 mm
   C. 75 mm
   D. 140 mm
   E. 115 mm
   REF: Ibid., p. 16

24. Suppressed plasma renin activity is seen in which one of the following conditions?
   A. Bartter's syndrome
   B. licorice ingestion
   C. oral contraceptives
   D. chronic diuretic use
   E. chronic potassium depletion
   REF: Berliner, R.W. and Orloff, J. (Eds.): *Handbook of Physiology, Section 8-Renal Physiology,* Williams and Wilkins, Baltimore, 1973, p. 866

25. Gordon's syndrome is characterized by hypertension, hyperkalemia, and expansion of the extracellular volume. Which one of the following is true?
   A. the condition is associated with cystic changes in the kidneys, spleen and liver
   B. plasma renin and aldosterone levels are high
   C. sodium reabsorption in the proximal tubules is increased
   D. delivery of sodium to the distal convoluted tubule is increased
   E. deformity of the nails and ears are common
   REF: Black, D. (Ed.): *Renal Disease, 3rd Ed.,* Blackwell Scientific Publications, Oxford, London, 1972, p. 89

26. Which of the following drugs stimulate renin release?
A. clonidine
B. chlorothiazide
C. reserpine
D. furosemide
E. propranolol
REF: Berliner, R.W. and Orloff, J. (Eds.): *Handbook of Physiology, Section 8-Renal Physiology,* Williams and Wilkins, Baltimore, 1973, p. 879

27. Which one of the following features is rare in medullary sponge kidney?
A. recurrent hematuria
B. recurrent nephrolithiasis
C. recurrent urinary tract infection
D. anemia
E. abnormal IVP
REF: Beeson, P.B., McDermott, W., Wyngaarden, J.B. (Eds.): *Cecil Textbook of Medicine, 15 Ed.,* W.B. Saunders Company, Philadelphia, 1979, p. 1455

28. Renal vein thrombosis may be a complication of all of the following EXCEPT
A. hypernephroma
B. congestive heart failure
C. terminally, with papillary necrosis
D. nephrosclerosis
E. nephrotic syndrome
REF: Thorne, G. et al. (Eds.): *Harrison's Principles of Internal Medicine, 8th Ed.,* McGraw-Hill Book Company, New York, 1977, p. 1458

29. Patients with proximal renal tubular acidosis will have an acid urine if
   A. serum bicarbonate is low
   B. serum chloride is low
   C. serum potassium is low
   D. serum sodium is low
   E. none of above
   REF: Maxwell, M.H. and Kleeman, C.R.: *Clinical Disorders of Fluid and Electrolyte Metabolism, 2nd Ed.*, McGraw-Hill Book Company, New York, 1972, p. 826

30. Streptococcal infection is followed by
   A. nephritis after a latent period of 18 days
   B. rheumatic fever after a latent period of 10 days
   C. nephritis after a latent period of 10 days
   D. a reduced incidence of nephritis with gamma globulin therapy
   E. rheumatic fever and nephritis, with a serologically similar organism
   REF: Pickering, G.: *High Pressure, 2nd Ed.*, Grune & Stratton, Inc., New York, 1968, p. 472

31. Which one of the following is helpful in distinguishing between poststreptococcal glomerulonephritis and benign essential hematuria (focal glomerulonephritis)?
   A. ASO titer
   B. urinary sediment
   C. throat swab culture
   D. proteinuria
   E. relationship of hematuria to infection of throat
   REF: Hamburger, J. et al. (Eds.): *Nephrology, Vol. 104,* Year Book Medical Publishers, Chicago, 1971-74, p. 962

32. All of the following are true in mesangiocapillary glomerulonephritis EXCEPT
    A. C3 levels are high
    B. C3 nephritic factor (C3NeF) is present in the serum
    C. C3 catabolism is accelerated
    D. C3 synthesis is depressed
    E. recurrent infections may occur
    REF: Ibid.
    Germuth, F.G. and Rodriguez, E.: *Immunopathology of the Renal Glomerulus*, Little, Brown and Company, Boston, 1973

33. Which one of the following qualitative tests for proteinuria is most sensitive?
    A. "shake test"
    B. dip stick
    C. heat and acetic acid
    D. sulfosalicylic acid
    E. Esbach's reagent
    REF: Papper, S.: *Clinical Nephrology, 2nd Ed.*, Little, Brown and Company, Boston, 1978, p. 11

34. Which one of the following gives false positive precipitation tests on urinalysis?
    A. aspirin
    B. high doses of tetracycline
    C. tolbutamide
    D. alpha-methyldopa
    E. Indomethacin
    REF: Eurley, L.E. and Gottschalk, C.W.: *Strauss and Welts' Diseases of the Kidney, 3rd Ed.*, Little, Brown and Company, Boston, 1979
    Black, D. (Ed.): *Renal Disease, 3rd Ed.*, Blackwell Scientific Publications, Oxford, London, 1972

35. A 17-year-old college student excretes 50 mg of protein/24 hour supine, and 950 mg upright. The correct approach to this problem would be to
   A. perform a renal biopsy
   B. order a pyelogram
   C. repeat the test in 12 months
   D. rule out obstructive uropathy by cystoscopy
   E. determine the selectivity of the proteinuria
   REF: Eurley, L.E. and Gottschalk, C.W.: *Strauss and Welts' Diseases of the Kidney, 3rd Ed.*, Little, Brown and Company, Boston, 1979, p. 70

36. Collections of electron-dense deposits between the basement membrane and the epithelial cells are seen most frequently in
   A. lipoid nephrosis
   B. diabetic glomerulosclerosis
   C. amyloidosis
   D. penicillamine nephropathy
   E. chronic tuberculosis
   REF: Ibid., p. 562

37. A 40-year-old man develops nephrotic syndrome, hypertension, hematuria and a rapidly increasing serum creatinine. Serum complement level is normal. The patient requires repeated dialysis, but after four months, the renal function levels off at a serum creatinine level of 5 mg/100 ml. The most likely diagnosis is
   A. acute poststreptococcal glomerulonephritis
   B. rapidly progressive extracapillary glomerulonephritis
   C. mesangiocapillary glomerulonephritis
   D. membranous glomerulopathy
   E. renal vein thrombosis
   REF: Ibid., pp. 712-714

Nephrology / 143

38. Cyclophosphamide in nephrotic syndrome has been of proven value in
   A. the remission of membranous glomerulonephritis
   B. relapsing steroid-sensitive syndrome due to minimal lesion type in childhood
   C. proliferative glomerulonephritis
   D. nephrotic syndrome of infancy
   E. hereditary nephritis
   REF: Black, D. (Ed.): *Renal Disease, 3rd Ed.*, Blackwell Scientific Publications, Oxford, London, 1972, p. 359

39. The bacterial population in the bladder is significantly increased by
   A. residual urine
   B. hydration
   C. frequent micturition
   D. quantity of IgA in urine
   E. none of the above
   REF: Ibid., pp. 386-387

40. Which one of the following is the most reliable evidence of acute renal parenchymal infection?
   A. leukocyte casts in urine
   B. bacteriuria more than 100,000/ml
   C. numerous WBC/HPF
   D. numerous renal epithelial cells
   E. renal biopsy
   REF: Ibid., p.404

41. All are true about xanthogranulomatous pyelonephritis EXCEPT
   A. profound weight loss
   B. *E. coli* is the most common organism
   C. there are lucent areas on nephrotomography
   D. it is associated with staghorn calculi
   E. radiologically it may mimic a tumor
   REF: Heptinstall, R.H.: *Pathology of the Kidney, 2nd. Ed.*, Little, Brown and Company, Boston, 1974, p. 916

42. Acute tubulointerstitial nephritis may in part be characterized by which one of the following?
    A. a hypersensitive reaction involving tubules and interstitial tissue rather than glomeruli
    B. most reports have implicated sulfonamides, methicillin or large doses of penicillin
    C. arteritis is not a feature but lesions are characterized by irregular interstitial accumulation of leukocytes containing many mononuclear cells
    D. hematuria with mild to moderate proteinuria is common
    E. abnormally low blood urea nitrogen
    REF: Thorne, G. et al. (Eds.): *Harrison's Principles of Internal Medicine, 8th Ed.*, McGraw-Hill Book Company, New York, 1977, p. 1478

43. Which one of the following is NOT a tubulointerstitial disease?
    A. analgesic nephropathy
    B. acute glomerulonephritis
    C. transplant rejection
    D. Balkan nephropathy
    E. Sjögren syndrome
    REF: Brenner, B.H. and Rector, F.C. (Eds.): *The Kidney*, W.B. Saunders Company, Philadelphia, 1976, p. 1114

44. Which of the following apply to renal tubular acidosis?
    A. in proximal RTA, during severe acidosis, bicarbonate disappears from the urine
    B. in distal RTA, during severe acidosis, bicarbonaturia persists
    C. distal RTA occurs characteristically in Fanconi's syndrome
    D. proximal RTA occurs in autoimmune disorders
    E. none of the above
    REF: Ibid., pp. 622–635

45. Which one of the following is diagnostic of hypokalemic nephropathy?
   A. lack of concentration ability after infusion of ADH and a serum K of 2 mEq/l
   B. loss of diluting capacity and serum K 2.5 mEq/l
   C. serum K 1.2 mEq/l
   D. serum K 3.5 mEq/l and glomerular sclerosis
   E. serum K 3.5 mEq/l and renal biopsy showing multiple vacuoles in the renal tubular epithelium
   REF: Beeson, P.B., McDermott, W., Wyngaarden, J.B. (Eds.): *Cecil Textbook of Medicine, 15th Ed.*, W.B. Saunders Company, Philadelphia, 1979, p. 1438

46. In hot climates which one of the following stones are frequently seen?
   A. cystine
   B. calcium oxalate
   C. uric acid
   D. magnesium phosphate
   E. triple phosphate
   REF: Maxwell, M.H. and Kleeman, C.R.: *Clinical Disorders of Fluid and Electrolyte Metabolism, 2nd Ed.*, McGraw-Hill Book Company, New York, 1972, p. 1099

47. Which one is the most important step of vitamin D metabolism carried out in the kidney?
   A. 25-hydroxylation of cholecalciferol
   B. 1-hydroxylation of 25-hydroxycholecalciferol
   C. production of dihydrotachysterol
   D. both 1- and 25-hydroxylation of cholecalciferol
   E. only ergocalciferol may be converted to 1, 25-hydroxycholecalciferol in the kidney
   REF: Black, D. (Ed.): *Renal Disease, 3rd Ed.*, Blackwell Scientific Publications, Oxford, London, 1972, p. 474

48. Magnesium ammonium phosphate stones are found in association with
   A. high magnesium intake
   B. high ammonium intake
   C. high phosphate intake
   D. infection with urea-splitting organisms
   E. prolonged excessive use of alkali
   REF: Eurley, L.E. and Gottchalk, C.W.: *Strauss and Welts' Diseases of the Kidney, 3rd Ed.*, Little, Brown and Company, Boston, 1979, pp. 921-923

49. A 30-year-old female presented with low back pain and urinary tract infection; IVP showed blunting of the minor calyces with ureteral dilatation. Which one of the following may be related to the patient's condition?
   A. vague frontal headaches for 10 years
   B. migrainous headaches for 5 years
   C. use of contraceptive pill for 10 years
   D. use of Pro-Banthine daily for 6 weeks for peptic ulcer
   E. history of herpes zoster 2 years earlier
   REF: Beeson, P.B., McDermott, W., Wyngaarden, J.B. (Eds.): *Cecil Textbook of Medicine, 15th Ed.*, W.B. Saunders Company, Philadelphia, 1979, pp. 223-224

50. All of the following have been implicated in inducing or activating SLE EXCEPT
   A. isoniazid
   B. Mesantoin
   C. procainamide
   D. phenytoin
   E. prednisone
   REF: Black, D. (Ed.): *Renal Disease, 3rd. Ed.*, Blackwell Scientific Publications, Oxford, London, 1972, pp. 607-608

51. Pulmonary hemorrhage with nephritis may be found in
    A. SLE
    B. polyarteritis nodosa
    C. Henoch-Schönlein syndrome
    D. Goodpasture's syndrome
    E. all of the above
    REF: Germuth, F.G. and Rodriguez, E.: *Immunopathology of the Renal Glomerulus*, Little, Brown and Company, Boston, 1973, p. 195

52. A 40-year-old male suffering from multiple myeloma for 6 months had been treated intensively with chemotherapy and was admitted to the hospital in a drowsy state. BUN 150 mg, Creatinine 10 mg., uric acid 12 mg, Na+ 132 mEq, K+ 5 mEq, Cl− 107, CO_2 16 mmol/l, urine output 300 cc/24 hours. After proper hydration and alkali therapy, urine output increased to 400 cc/24 hours. IV mannitol (50 gm) was given without any appreciable effect. Which of the following should be done immediately?
    A. IV furosemide 500 mg
    B. allopurinol 100 mg q.i.d. PO
    C. IV acetazolamide 250 mg
    D. peritoneal dialysis
    E. mannitol 100 gm IV
    REF: Beeson, P.B., McDermott, W., Wyngaarden, J.B. (Eds.): *Cecil Textbook of Medicine, 15th Ed.*, W.B. Saunders Company, Philadelphia, 1979, p. 1405

53. The most frequent cause of death in acute renal failure is
    A. uremia
    B. pulmonary edema
    C. hyperkalemia
    D. infection
    E. hyponatremia
    REF: Schrier, R.W. (Ed.): *Renal and Electrolyte Disorders.* Little, Brown and Company, Boston, 1976, p. 312

54. Which one of the following statements is FALSE?
A. the digoxin dose in most uremic patients is 0.125 mg on alternate days
B. the dose of procainamide in uremia is unchanged
C. for propranolol, little dose modification is required in uremia
D. lidocaine in uremia is given in normal doses
E. the dose of quinidine in uremia is unchanged
REF: Anderson, R.J., et al.: *Clinical Use of Drugs in Renal Failure*, Charles C Thomas, Springfield, Ill., 1978, pp. 159-168

55. Which one of the following does NOT play a part in the pathogenesis of renal osteodystrophy?
A. parathormone suppression
B. resistance to vitamin D
C. calcium malabsorption
D. hyperphosphatemia
E. metabolic acidosis
REF: Eurley, L.E. and Gottschalk, C.W.: *Strauss and Welts' Diseases of the Kidney, 3rd Ed.*, Little, Brown and Company, Boston, 1979, p. 313

56. Which one of the following doses is incorrect in a patient with a creatinine clearance of 5 ml/min?
A. ampicillin 500 mg bid
B. gentamicin 15 mg 8 hourly
C. cephalothin 0.5 gm bid
D. chloramphenicol 250 mg qid
E. carbenicillin 5 gm 4 hourly
REF: Anderson, R.J., et al.: *Clinical Use of Drugs in Renal Failure*, Charles C Thomas, Springfield, Ill., 1978, pp. 32-33

57. The average BUN in pregnancy is
A. 3 mg/dl
B. 9 mg/dl
C. 14 mg/dl
D. 20 mg/dl
E. 24 mg/dl
REF: Papper, S.: *Clinical Nephrology, 2nd Ed.*, Little, Brown and Company, Boston, 1978, p. 382

58. Essential hypertension rather than toxemia of pregnancy is more likely if
   A. the hypertension appears after 28 weeks
   B. the patient is a primipara
   C. proteinuria and edema are present
   D. the serum uric acid is normal
   E. the blood pressure was normal between pregnancies
   REF: Schrier, R.W. (Ed.): *Renal and Electrolyte Disorders,* Little, Brown and Company, Boston, 1976, p. 384

59. Systemic infections associated with immune-deposit nephritis are LEAST likely in which one of the following conditions?
   A. a five-year-old child with heavy proteinuria, edema, lipiduria and absence of hypertension
   B. the development of nephrotic syndrome in an East-African man who has had recurrent episodes of fever and chills
   C. hematuria and edema in a twenty-year-old woman with a nonpruritic rash, most marked on the palms and soles
   D. following surgery to correct obstructive hydrocephalus
   E. proteinuria and edema in a heroin addict
   REF: Eurley, L.E. and Gottschalk, C.W.: *Strauss and Welts', Diseases of the Kidney, 3rd Ed.,* Little, Brown and Company, Boston, 1979, pp. 661-662

60. Nephrectomy prior to transplantation should be performed in all of the following EXCEPT
   A. polycystic kidney disease with hemorrhage
   B. Wilms' tumor
   C. Goodpasture's syndrome
   D. Alport's syndrome
   E. persistent pyelonephritis
   REF: Becker, E.L., (Ed.): *Seminars in Nephrology,* John Wiley & Sons, Inc., New York, 1977, p. 1807

DIRECTIONS: Indicate whether each of the following statements is **True** or **False**.

61. Infantile polycystic kidney disease is sex-linked recessive.
62. Adult polycystic kidney is autosomal recessive.
63. Adult polycystic kidney is more common in men.
64. Hypertension is rare in polycystic disease.
65. Cardiac failure is a frequent cause of death.
    REF: De Wardner, H.E.: *The Kidney: An Outline of Normal and Abnormal Structure and Function, 4th Ed.*, Longman, Inc., New York, 1973, p. 401

DIRECTIONS: For Questions 66 through 70, match the numbered item with the **ONE** most appropriate lettered item.

66. Nitroprusside
67. Trimethapan
68. Methyldopa
69. Alpha-methylparatyrosine
70. Phenoxbenzamine

A. Increased venous capacitance
B. CNS action
C. Ganglionic blocker
D. Inhibits tyrosine
E. Alpha-adrenergic blockade
   REF: Genest, J.: *Hypertension,* McGraw-Hill Book Company, New York, 1977, p. 990

VIII: Gastroenterology

DIRECTIONS: Each of the questions or incomplete statements below is followed by five suggested answers or completions. Select the **one** that is **BEST** in each case.

1. Aluminum-containing antacids may be expected to
   A. interfere with fluoride absorption
   B. interfere with phosphorus absorption
   C. result in hypercalcuria
   D. result in all of the above
   E. result in none of the above
   REF: Gastroenterology 76:603, 1979

2. All of the following are relatively uncommon reasons for operative intervention in Crohn's disease of the colon EXCEPT
   A. anal stricture
   B. unremitting liver disease
   C. colonic obstruction
   D. perforations
   E. unremitting hemorrhage
   REF: Gastroenterology 76:607, 1979

3. Hyperthyroidism with associated malabsorption and diarrhea may be related to all of the following EXCEPT
   A. increased gastrointestinal transit
   B. rapid gastric emptying
   C. depressed pancreatic enzyme secretion
   D. all of the above
   E. none of the above
   REF: Am. J. Dig. Dis. 23:1003, 1978

4. Which of the following has not been identified as an effect of estrogens on the liver?
   A. cholesterol gallstone production
   B. diminished bile flow
   C. diminished BSP secretion
   D. pigment gallstone production
   E. development of hepatic adenomas
   REF: Gastroenterology 75:512, 1978

5. The probable pathogenesis of pseudomembranous colitis with the following antibiotics is
   A. direct cytotoxicity reaction caused by the drug
   B. direct cytotoxicity reaction caused by metabolites of the drugs
   C. cytotoxicity reaction caused by immune sensitivity to the drug
   D. cytotoxicity secondary to overgrowth of *Clostridia* in the antibiotic-treated gut
   E. none of the above
   REF: N. Engl. J. Med. 289:531, 1978

6. Which of the following is the most ominous criterion for the prediction of fatality from peptic ulcer disease?
   A. solitary gastric ulcer
   B. solitary duodenal ulcer
   C. combined gastric and duodenal ulcer
   D. diagnosis before age 50
   E. prediagnostic symptoms present for more than one year
   REF: Gastroenterology 75:1055, 1978

7. All of the following are relative contraindications to percutaneous liver biopsy EXCEPT
   A. fever
   B. ascites
   C. anemia with hemoglobin less than 9.5 gm/dl
   D. performance on an outpatient basis
   E. prothrombin times less than 50% of the normal activity
   REF: Gastroenterology 74:103, 1978

8. In dealing with patients exposed to parenteral inoculation with hepatitis B, the most appropriate approach would be
   A. administration of immune serum globulin of the standard or pooled variety
   B. administration of hepatitis B immune globulin
   C. no prophylaxis is necessary but serial SGOTs should be drawn
   D. no prophylaxis is necessary, and no further follow-up is necessary unless jaundice appears
   E. none of the above
   REF: Ann. Intern. Med. 88:285, 1978

9. Nonoperative management of pancreatic ascites secondary to internal fistula includes
   A. acetazolamide
   B. atropine
   C. hyperalimentation
   D. chest tube
   E. all of the above
   REF: Gastroenterology 74:134, 1978

10. Which of the following has been demonstrated to be of significant benefit in the medical therapy of acute pancreatitis?
    A. nasogastric suction
    B. aprotinin
    C. anticholinergics
    D. glucagon
    E. none of the above
    REF: Gastroenterology 74:620, 1978

11. Carcinoembryonic antigen assay (CEA) of pleural effusion and ascitic fluid has
    A. been substantially better than cytologic studies for detecting malignant effusions
    B. been substantially less effective than cytologic studies for detecting malignant effusions
    C. been of about the same value as cytologic studies for the detection of malignant effusions
    D. a sensitivity about the same as cytologic studies but often is positive, when cytology is not positive or vice versa, making the use of both studies additive in the overall evaluation for maligant effusions
    E. none of the above
    REF: Ann. Intern. Med. 88:635, 1978

12. Lactase levels fall to low (adult) levels in white children at about age
    A. 3
    B. 5
    C. 7
    D. 9
    E. 11+
    REF: Gastroenterology 75:847, 1978

13. The frequency of HLA B13 histocompatibility antigen in alcoholics with cirrhosis is
    A. higher than in normals
    B. higher than in alcoholics without cirrhosis
    C. higher than both normals and alcoholics without cirrhosis
    D. higher than normals but the same as in alcoholics without cirrhosis
    E. the same as in normals but lower than alcoholics without cirrhosis
    REF: Gut 20:288, 1979

14. In patients with primary biliary cirrhosis, the laboratory study that shows the closest correlation with progression of the disease is
    A. serum transaminase
    B. phosphatase
    C. bilirubin
    D. serum cholesterol
    E. antimitochondrial antibodies
    REF: Gut 20:137, 1979

15. Enteral hyperalimentation offers many practical advantages over parenteral approaches to hyperalimentation. The most common complication of enteral hyperalimentation is
    A. mechanical plugging of the tube
    B. hyperglycemia
    C. congestive heart failure
    D. diarrhea and cramping
    E. edema
    REF: Ann. Intern. Med. 90:63, 1979

16. With regard to hepatocellular carcinoma in the United States, which of the following statements is most correct?
    A. most patients will have serologic or tissue markers of hepatitis B virus infection
    B. patients with alcoholic liver disease preceding the hepatocellular carcinoma have evidence of hepatitis B infection as frequently as patients with nonalcoholic liver disease
    C. patients with hepatocellular carcinoma arising in normal liver frequently have evidence of hepatitis B virus infection
    D. patients with nonalcoholic chronic active liver disease have a very high incidence of hepatitis B virus infection
    E. all of the above
    REF: Gastroenterology 76:279, 1979

17. Which of the following may be associated with flat villous lesions on small biopsy?
    A. kwashiorkor
    B. acute infectious enteritis
    C. dermatitis herpetiformis
    D. neomycin enteropathy
    E. all of the above
    REF: Gastroenterology 76:375, 1979

18. With ethanol ingestion, which of the following GI effects may be related to intestinal absorption?
    A. increased gastric emptying time
    B. increased transit time
    C. decreased biliary secretion in chronic alcoholics
    D. increased pancreatic secretion with an acute dose of alcohol
    E. increased splanchnic circulation
    REF: Gastroenterology 76:388, 1979

19. Which of the following is regularly associated with upper esophageal sphincter dysfunction?
    A. Parkinson's disease
    B. myasthenia gravis
    C. thyrotoxicosis
    D. Huntington's chorea
    E. all of the above
    REF: Am. J. Dig. Dis. 23:275, 1978

20. All of the following symptoms and signs may be expected in patients with amoebic liver abscess. All may be expected in 80% or more of the patients with amoebic liver abscess EXCEPT
    A. abdominal pain
    B. tender hepatomegaly
    C. abnormal right-chest findings
    D. anorexia
    E. fever
    REF: Am. J. Dig. Dis. 23:110, 1978

21. The most common association between drug ingestion and acute pancreatitis would seem to be in those patients who are taking
    A. digitalis preparations
    B. corticosteroid preparations
    C. oral contraceptives
    D. diuretics
    E. antidepressant drugs
    REF: Lancet I:706, 1978

22. The prevention of travelers' diarrhea is most effective if one
    A. drinks only bottled water
    B. avoids all fresh fruits and vegetables
    C. takes 100 mg of doxycycline daily
    D. takes a single tablet of Lomotil twice daily
    E. none of the above
    REF: N. Engl. J. Med. 298:758, 1978

23. The principal cause of malnutrition and nutritional deficiencies in liver disease is
    A. impairment of digestion and absorption
    B. failure of dietary intake
    C. alterations in hepatic metabolism of protein, carbohydrates, lipids, and other nutritional elements
    D. increased requirements secondary to hepatic alterations
    E. failure of storage function in the liver
    REF: Gastroenterology 74:770, 1978

24. Crohn's disease in the young presents primarily as
    A. ileocolitis
    B. colitis
    C. diffuse small bowel disease
    D. terminal ileal disease
    E. extraintestinal manifestations
    REF: Gastroenterology 74:807, 1978

25. Ultrasonic cholangiography is most useful in the differential diagnosis of cholestatic jaundice
    A. when the bilirubin is less than 10 mg/dl
    B. early in extrahepatic obstruction
    C. late in extrahepatic obstruction
    D. in differentiating malignant from nonmalignant extrahepatic obstruction
    E. postcholecystectomy
    REF: Ann. Intern. Med. 89:61, 1978

26. In the prospective follow-up of patients with chronic ulcerative colitis, which of the following would be the most significant factor with regard to malignant change?
    A. age of the patient
    B. duration of the patient's chronic ulcerative colitis
    C. extent of colonic involvement
    D. the appearance of the barium enema
    E. the presence of dysplasias in a colon biopsy
    REF: Gastroenterology 76:1, 1979

27. Patients less than 30 years old differ from older patients with idiopathic hemochromatosis in the frequency of
    A. diabetes mellitus
    B. liver involvement
    C. skin pigmentation
    D. cardiomyopathy
    E. all of the above
    REF: Gastroenterology 76:178, 1979

28. Malabsorption syndrome as a result of bacterial overgrowth usually will affect
    A. fat
    B. carbohydrates
    C. protein
    D. vitamin B_{12}
    E. all of the above
    REF: Gastroenterology 76:1035, 1979

29. Anastomotic ulcers that develop after gastric resection for acid peptic disease are most effectively treated by
    A. surgical revision of the anastomosis
    B. intensive antacid therapy
    C. the use of H₂ blocking agents
    D. vagotomy
    E. anticholinergics
    REF: Gastroenterology 76:82, 1979

30. All of the following are associated with a defect in biliary secretion of lipid EXCEPT
    A. hypercholesterolemia
    B. spur or burr cells
    C. xanthoma
    D. increased lipoprotein X
    E. steatorrhea
    REF: Viewpoint Dig. Dis. 10:1, 1978

31. The principal hormonal control of contraction of gallbladder rests with
    A. cholecystokinin
    B. vasoactive intestinal peptide (VIP)
    C. secretin
    D. gastrin
    E. heteroglucagon
    REF: Viewpoint Dig. Dis. 11:3, 1979

32. Generally speaking, lactase-deficient individuals are capable of tolerating
    A. one glass of milk a day
    B. two glasses of milk a day
    C. three glasses of milk a day
    D. four glasses of milk a day
    E. five glasses of milk a day
    REF: Gastroenterology 74:44, 1978

33. If individuals with cirrhotic portal hypertension secondary to alcoholism continue to drink, they are more likely than those who stopped drinking to present in the hospital with
    A. recurrent variceal hemorrhage
    B. ascites
    C. encephalopathy
    D. jaundice
    E. all of the above
    REF: Gastroenterology 74:64, 1978

34. The treatment of severe acute alcoholic hepatitis should include
    A. steroids
    B. avoidance of steroids
    C. forced feeding
    D. intravenous hyperalimentation
    E. none of the above
    REF: Gastroenterology 75:193, 1978

35. Patients with reflux esophagitis may have demonstrated sensitivity to
    A. Zero 1N hydrochloric acid
    B. orange juice
    C. orange juice adjusted to pH 7
    D. coffee
    E. all of the above
    REF: Gastroenterology 75:240, 1978

36. The upper esophageal sphincter responds by contracting in the presence of
    A. normal saline
    B. twice normal saline
    C. triple normal saline
    D. tenth normal hydrochloric acid
    E. all of the above
    REF: Gastroenterology 75:268, 1978

37. In individuals with a history of rectal bleeding, negative conventional barium enemas, and negative proctosigmoidoscopies, colonoscopy can be expected to provide a diagnosis in
   A. 10% of the patients
   B. 20% of the patients
   C. 40% of the patients
   D. 75% of the patients
   E. 90% of the patients
   REF: Ann. Intern. Med. 89:907, 1978

38. When the prevalence of diverticular disease of the colon is examined, one finds
   A. a prevalence in patients recovering from myocardial infarction that is higher than that among matched control subjects
   B. a prevalence in matched control subjects that is the same as that among infarct patients
   C. a prevalence in control subjects higher than that found in postinfarct patients
   D. an incidence among patients with premature ventricular contractions that is higher than that among controls
   E. none of the above
   REF: Gut 19:1054, 1978

39. The most common form of clinical presentation in Wilson's Disease is
   A. neurologic disease
   B. psychiatric disease
   C. hepatic disease
   D. hemolytic anemia
   E. bone disease
   REF: N. Engl. J. Med. 298:1347, 1978

40. Follow-up studies after simple suture closure of perforated duodenal ulcers have shown the procedure
    A. is well tolerated with half the patients remaining free of symptoms for at least a ten-year period
    B. is poorly tolerated by those patients who had preperforation symptoms
    C. is well tolerated by those patients with preperforation symptoms but poorly tolerated by individuals who had been symptom free until the time of perforation
    D. is inadequate as definitive therapy and requires a second procedure at a later date
    E. should always be accompanied by definitive procedure at the time of initial surgery unless local factors make this overwhelmingly complicated
    REF: Lancet II:749, 1978

41. All of the following are associated with risk factors in the development of cholesterol gallstones EXCEPT
    A. clofibrate therapy
    B. terminal ileal disease
    C. oral contraceptives
    D. alcoholic cirrhosis
    E. American Indian ancestry
    REF: N. Engl. J. Med. 299:1221, 1978

42. The average incubation period for hepatitis B is about two months based on the appearance of abnormal SGOT levels. With regard to hepatitis B surface antigen, which of the following is correct?
    A. it is detectable at about the same time the transaminase becomes detectable
    B. it is detectable in the circulation several weeks before the transaminase becomes detectable
    C. it is detectable often as early as one or two weeks after exposure and months before the transaminase rises
    D. it has usually disappeared by the time the transaminase goes up
    E. none of the above
    REF: N. Engl. J. Med. 300:100, 1979

43. In individuals with chronic alcoholic pancreatitis, one would expect to find clinically significant evidence of alcoholic liver disease in
 A. 10%
 B. 20%
 C. 40%
 D. 70%
 E. 100%
 REF: Am. J. Dig. Dis. 23:618, 1978

44. Pulmonary edema has been found to occur in approximately a third of the patients with fulminant hepatic failure. Its occurrence seems related to
 A. renal failure
 B. elevated pulmonary wedge pressure
 C. clinical evidence of left heart failure
 D. all of the above
 E. none of the above
 REF: Gastroenterology 74:859, 1978

45. Maintenance therapy with cimetidine in the treatment of peptic ulcer has been found to
 A. be ineffective because of failure of drug action after several months of administration
 B. be severely limited by the frequent toxic side effects of long-term cimetidine administration
 C. significantly reduce the recurrence of ulcer
 D. have no effect on the recurrence of peptic ulcer
 E. none of the above
 REF: Lancet I:403, 1978

46. Ten years after the onset of chronic ulcerative colitis one would expect to find
    A. extension of the disease in over half of the patients
    B. that the patient has a substantial risk of development of carcinoma in that ten-year interval
    C. that patients, particularly with extensive colitis, are more likely than not to require surgical therapy
    D. that the involvement that is known as ulcerative proctitis is unlikely to require either hospitalization or operation in that interval
    E. all of the above
    REF: Lancet I:1140, 1978

DIRECTIONS: For each of the following questions or incomplete statements, ONE or MORE of the answers or completions given is correct. Select:
   A if only 1, 2 and 3 are correct,
   B if only 1 and 3 are correct,
   C if only 2 and 4 are correct,
   D if only 4 is correct,
   E if all are correct.

---

47. Treatment with chenodeoxycholic acid to dissolve gallstones may be expected to produce which of the following changes?
    1. elevation of bilirubin
    2. elevation of cholesterol
    3. elevation of triglycerides
    4. elevation in SGPT
    REF: Gastroenterology 75:1016, 1978

48. The drug of choice for medical dissolution of cholesterol gallstones appear, at least this time, to be
    1. heparin
    2. chenodoxycholic acid
    3. bran
    4. ursodeoxycholic acid
    REF: Lancet II:367, 1977

49. Noncholera *Vibrio* infections have been associated with which of the following vehicles?
   1. sea water
   2. egg salad
   3. shellfish
   4. well water
   REF: Ann. Intern. Med. 88:602, 1978

50. Intestinal bypass operations for obesity have been associated with
   1. malabsorption of medications, most specifically thyroid replacement with the production of hypothyroidism
   2. significant renal damage secondary to oxalate deposition in the kidney
   3. copper deficiency significant enough to produce leukopenia
   4. immune complex disease
   REF: Ann. Intern. Med. 89:594, 1978
   　　　Ann. Intern. Med. 90:941, 1979
   　　　Ann. Intern. Med. 89:491, 1978

51. Intoxication to the degree that will produce serum alcohol levels above 70 mg/dl will result in which of the following changes in esophageal function?
   1. fall in the lower esophageal sphincter's pressure
   2. decrease in the force of esophageal peristaltic wave
   3. decrease in the velocity of the esophageal peristaltic wave
   4. reduction in the lower esophageal sphincter pressure response to pantagastrin or a protein meal
   REF: Gastroenterology 75:1133, 1978

Directions Summarized				
A	B	C	D	E
1, 2, 3 only	1, 3 only	2, 4 only	4 only	All are correct

52. A trial of low-dose (7.5 mg/day) prednisone therapy to prevent relapse in Crohn's disease has shown that
    1. the relapse rate was not improved
    2. there was no alteration in the frequency with which extension of disease occurred
    3. the radiologic recurrence rate was the same for both prednisone-treated and control patients
    4. even at this dose, steroids were not tolerated, and patients had to be withdrawn from therapy because of side effects
    REF: Gut 19:606, 1978

53. Veno-occlusive disease of the liver is known to be associated with
    1. plant toxins
    2. allogeneic bone marrow transplantation
    3. immunosuppresive agents
    4. hepatitis A virus
    REF: Ann. Intern. Med. 90:158, 1979

54. Gastric emptying rates have been shown to be
    1. inversely related to body surface area
    2. directly related to body surface area
    3. inversely related to body weight
    4. directly related to body weight
    REF: Gastroenterology 74:1258, 1978

55. Which of the following might be incriminated etiologically in secondary intestinal pseudo-obstruction?
    1. hyperparathyroidism
    2. nontropical sprue
    3. tricyclic antidepressants
    4. jejunal diverticulosis
    REF: Gastroenterology 74:922, 1978

56. Postvagotomy diarrhea
    1. is worsened if the patient also has had a cholecystectomy
    2. tends to respond to propranolol
    3. will improve with bile-acid binding particularly in those individuals who also have cholecystectomy
    4. is markedly improved by a course of aluminum hydroxide gel

    REF: Lancet I:635, 1978

57. In Peutz-Jeghers syndrome, which of the following extra-intestinal manifestations have been regularly observed?
    1. mandibular osteomas
    2. dental cysts
    3. desmoid tumors in abdominal wall scars
    4. thyroid cancer

    REF: Gastroenterology 74:1325, 1978

58. The diagnosis of achalasia of the esophagus should be based upon typical
    1. clinical features of dysphagia
    2. radiologic features of esophageal dilation and "beaking"
    3. manometric features with aperistalsis in the esophageal body and a hypertensive esophageal sphincter
    4. features on upper endoscopy

    REF: Ann. Intern. Med. 89:315, 1978

59. Following successful treatment of *Giardia* infection, one would expect to observe
    1. an improvement in D-xylose tolerance
    2. an improvement in vitamin B_{12} absorption
    3. a fall in fecal fats
    4. an improvement in intestinal lactase levels

    REF: Gastroenterology 77:61, 1979

Directions Summarized

A	B	C	D	E
1, 2, 3 only	1, 3 only	2, 4 only	4 only	All are correct

60. An attempt to dissolve cholesterol gallstones by the administration of chenodoxycholic acid may be associated with
  1. elevated serum SGOT
  2. elevated serum alkaline phosphatase
  3. elevated serum levels of indirect reacting bilirubin
  4. depressed hemoglobin levels
  REF: Gastroenterology 77:121, 1979

61. The presence of circulating immune complexes in the course of hepatitis B infection may be associated with the production of
  1. hepatic encephalopathy
  2. urticaria
  3. jaundice
  4. glomerulonephritis
  REF: Ann. Intern. Med. 89:34, 1978

62. Ethanol ingestion has been associated with
  1. hypoglycemia
  2. hyperuricemia
  3. hyperlipidemia
  4. thrombocytopenia
  REF: Viewpoints Dig. Dis. 11:2, 1979

63. In patients with dermatitis herpetiformis given a gluten-free diet, one would expect
    1. both skin and jejunal lesions to be present and improve
    2. skin lesions present but jejunal lesions absent with improvement in the skin
    3. skin and jejunal lesions present and after therapy improvement in the jejunal lesions but not in the skin
    4. skin and jejunal lesions present with neither responding to the diet
    REF: Gut 19:754, 1978

64. In the treatment of gastric ulcer, a recurrence is more likely if the
    1. ulcer is unhealed at the time of discharge
    2. patient is male
    3. patient is over age 60
    4. patient smokes
    REF: Gut 19:419, 1978

65. Serum gastrin levels are found to be significantly increased
    1. in Cushing's syndrome
    2. with short-term glucocorticoid administration
    3. with long-term glucocorticoid administration
    4. with a single dose of intravenously administered glucocorticoids
    REF: Gut 19:10, 1978

66. In the idiopathic intestinal pseudo-obstruction syndrome secondary to visceral myopathy, which of the following organs is (are) usually involved?
    1. duodenum
    2. ilium
    3. colon
    4. urinary bladder
    REF: Ann. Intern. Med. 89:600, 1978

Directions Summarized				
A	B	C	D	E
1, 2, 3 only	1, 3 only	2, 4 only	4 only	All are correct

67. Islet-cell tumors of the pancreas have been found to excrete which of the following hormones?
    1. gastrin
    2. insulin
    3. glucagon
    4. somatostatin
    REF: Ann. Intern. Med. 90:817, 1979

68. Diabetic gastroenteropathy may include
    1. decrease in esophageal peristalsis and the lower esophageal sphincter pressure
    2. delayed gastric emptying
    3. diarrhea
    4. constipation
    REF: Gut 19:1153, 1978

69. Recent colonoscopic studies indicate that colonic adenomas over 1 cm are predominately
    1. left sided
    2. missed by barium enema
    3. in the sigmoid colon
    4. multiple rather than single
    REF: Gut 20:240, 1979

70. Replacement therapy with pancreatic enzyme is
    1. substantially improved by the use of enteric-coated enzyme
    2. not improved by any of these maneuvers
    3. substantially improved by the use of supplemental antacids
    4. substantially improved by the use of cimetidine
    REF: N. Engl. J. Med. 297:854, 1977

71. The development of gastrointestinal symptoms presenting as bloody diarrhea would suggest pseudomembranous enterocolitis as a diagnosis if the patient was taking which of the following drugs?
    1. clindamycin
    2. tetracycline
    3. lincomycin
    4. ampicillin
    REF: Lancet II:707, 1978

72. Patients with gastroesophageal reflux treated with cimetidine experience
    1. little symptomatic relief
    2. marked symptomatic improvement
    3. prompt healing of associated esophagitis
    4. no change in acid sensitivity of the esophageal mucosa when measured by perfusion test
    REF: Lancet II:1068, 1978

73. *Giardia* infection has been associated with
    1. fat malabsorption
    2. IgA deficiency
    3. trophozoite penetration of the mucosa
    4. biliary tract dysfunction
    REF: Am. J. Dig. Dis. 23:559, 1978

74. Esophageal motor dysfunction in elderly patients is most likely to be caused by
    1. smooth muscle atrophy
    2. acid peptic reflux
    3. dental deterioration
    4. decrease in the number of ganglion cells in Auerbach's plexus
    REF: Am. J. Dig. Dis. 23:443, 1978

	Directions Summarized			
A	B	C	D	E
1, 2, 3 only	1, 3 only	2, 4 only	4 only	All are correct

75. In the treatment of Menétrièr's disease with associated peripheral edema secondary to gastric protein loss treatment, which of the following drugs has been found to decrease the gastric protein leakage?
    1. anticholinergics
    2. prostaglandin derivatives
    3. H_2 receptor blockers
    4. antacids
    REF: Gastroenterology 74:903, 1978

IX: Pulmonary

DIRECTIONS: Each of the questions or incomplete statements below is followed by suggested answers or completions. Select the **BEST** answer(s) in each case.

---

1. A 34-year-old West Virginia hunter is seen with a fever of 103° F and severe retrosternal pain worsened by coughing and eased by sitting forward. He has a small ulcer on his hand and some axillary node enlargement. Physical examination shows evidence of a right upper lobe pneumonia and in addition a definite pericardial rub is heard. He has leucocytosis. Examination of his sputum shows scanty gram-negative bacilli. The antibiotic regimen of choice is
   A. streptomycin and chloramphenicol
   B. ampicillin
   C. novobiocin
   D. penicillin
   E. erythromycin
   REF: Baum, G.L. (Ed.): *Textbook of Pulmonary Diseases,* *2nd Ed.*, Little, Brown and Company, Boston, 1974, Chapter 7

2. A 5-year-old child develops chickenpox. The illness is severe and two weeks later he becomes febrile again and develops a productive cough. Physical examination reveals a few scattered rhonchi and some basal rales (crepitations). Chest film shows patchy infiltrates in both mid and lower zones. Which of the following organisms is most likely to be the etiological agent?
A. *Haemophilus influenzae*
B. Varicella virus
C. Alpha-hemolytic streptococcus
D. *Staphylococcus aureus*
E. Bacteroides
REF: Kendig, E.L.: *Disorders of the Respiratory Tract in Children, Vol. 1*, Pulmonary Disorders, W.B. Saunders Company, Philadelphia, 1972, Chapter 49

3. The diagnosis of infection with *A. fumigatus* depends upon which of the following?
A. repeated cultures of the organism from trachea
B. positive serum precipitin reaction for *A. fumigatus*
C. an immediate skin reaction (type I) to aspergillus antigen
D. a delayed skin reaction (type III) to aspergillus antigen
E. finding of Curshmann's spirals on sputum examination
REF: Baum, G.L. (Ed.): *Textbook of Pulmonary Diseases, 2nd Ed.*, Little, Brown and Company, Boston, 1974, Chapter 10

4. A 4-year-old boy was seen with anorexia, low grade fever and recurrent attacks of "bronchitis". Physical examination revealed painful muscles and joints, and marked hepatomegaly. Examination of the fundi revealed with appeared to be a retinal tumor. The parasite probably responsible for this disease is
A. *Fasciola hepatica*
B. *Ascaris lumbricoides*
C. *Toxocara canis*
D. *Trichinella spiralis*
E. *Taenia solium*
REF: Kendig, E.L.: *Disorders of the Respiratory Tract in Children, Vol. 1*, Pulmonary Disorders, W.B. Saunders Company, Philadelphia, 1972, p. 763

5. Which of the following organisms is the most common pathogen isolated from patients with cystic fibrosis?
   A. *Neisseria gonorrhoeae*
   B. *Streptococcus faecalis*
   C. *Staphylococcus epidermidis*
   D. *Diplococcus pneumoniae*
   E. *Escherichia coli*
   F. *Staphylococcus aureus*
   G. *Pseudomonas pseudomallei*
   REF: Ibid., Chapter 38

6. In which of the following trades does an increased risk of tuberculosis occur?
   A. coal mining
   B. knife grinding
   C. gold mining
   D. tin smelting
   E. textile workers
   REF: Morgan, W.K.C. and Seaton, A.: *Occupational Lung Diseases*, W.B. Saunders Company, Philadelphia, 1975, Chapter 17

7. A 47-year-old former iron ore miner, now employed as a custodian, is observed to have a 3 cm shadow at the right apex on a background of small regular shadows. The radiographic appearances have not changed for the past three years, yet on a routine sputum examination, a few scanty, acid-fast bacilli are observed. His PPD test is 6 mm. He lives with his wife and his only child has now left home. What is the next step?
   A. admit patient to hospital and start on INH, rifampin and ethambutol
   B. start patient on INH alone
   C. tell the patient to stop working and start on INH, rifampin and ethambutol as an out patient
   D. send further smears, await cultures of the original and the additional specimens and delay any decision until the cultures are available
   REF: Ibid., Chapter 17

8. The original culture grows out colonies of acid-fast bacilli in 5 days. These have an unusual, somewhat beaded appearance. A subsequent smear and culture yields similar findings. The bacillus could be which of the following?
A. *M. tuberculosis*
B. *M. phlei*
C. *M. xenopi*
D. *M. kansasii*
E. *M. fortuitum*
REF: Baum, G.L. (Ed.): *Textbook of Pulmonary Diseases*, 2nd Ed., Little, Brown and Company, Boston, 1974, Chapter 13

9. Which of the following drug combinations should be avoided if possible in the treatment of tuberculosis?
A. PAS and streptomycin
B. PAS and INH
C. streptomycin and viomycin
D. pyrazinamide and PAS
E. PAS and ethionamide
F. viomycin and INH
REF: Ibid., Chapter 12
Crofton, J. and Douglas, A.: *Respiratory Diseases*, 2nd Ed., J.B. Lippincott, Philadelphia, 1975, Chapter 5

10. A 47-year-old man is found on a routine chest film to have a rounded 1.5 cm lesion in the medial segment of the right middle lobe. He has neither signs nor symptoms. He has smoked 30 cigarettes a day for 30 years. Bronchoscopy and sputum cytology are negative. His histoplasmin skin test shows 18 mm of induration and his tuberculin (PPD) 9 mm. The next step should be
A. to obtain complement fixation test for histoplasmosis
B. to repeat chest film in 3 months
C. thoracotomy and removal of right middle lobe
D. right scalene node biopsy
E. put patient on INH for 6 months and obtain chest radiographs at monthly intervals
REF: Baum, G.L. (Ed.): *Textbook of Pulmonary Diseases*, 2nd Ed., Little, Brown and Company, Boston, 1974, p. 781

11. Which of the following are absolute contraindications to surgery in lung cancer?
   A. paralysis of a vocal cord
   B. diaphragmatic paralysis due to an upper lobe tumor
   C. Eaton-Lambert syndrome
   D. gynecomastia
   E. pleural effusion
   REF: Ibid., Chapter 35
       Crofton, J. and Douglas, A.: *Respiratory Diseases, 2nd Ed.*, J.B. Lippincott, Philadelphia, 1975, Chapter 31

12. Which of the following complications of lung cancer indicate inoperability?
   A. the angiographic demonstration of complete blockage of the left pulmonary artery
   B. left recurrent laryngeal paralysis
   C. pleural effusion
   D. paralysis of the diaphragm by a lesion situated just above the left hilum
   REF: Baum, G.L. (Ed.): *Textbook of Pulmonary Diseases, 2nd Ed.*, Little, Brown and Company, Boston, 1974, Chapter 35
       Perry, K.M.A. and Sellors, T.H.: *Chest Diseases, Vol. 2*, Butterworth Company, Washington, D.C., 1963, Chapter 28

13. Biopsy of scalene nodes in suspected lung cancer is likely to yield a positive diagnosis under which of the following circumstances?
   A. hilar growths
   B. superior vena cava obstruction
   C. presence of palpable nodes in either supraclavicular fossa
   D. suspected oat cell carcinoma
   E. recurrent laryngeal palsy
   REF: Baum, G.L. (Ed.): *Textbook of Pulmonary Diseases, 2nd Ed.*, Little, Brown and Company, Boston, 1974, Chapter 35

178 / Pulmonary

14. A 74-year-old man has been shown to have a recurrent pleural effusion secondary to metastases from lung cancer. He can only be kept comfortable by repeated pleural taps at four to five day intervals. The treatment of choice is
   A. instillations of radioactive gold into the pleural cavity
   B. palliative radiotherapy with cobalt source to primary lesion (1500 r)
   C. decortication and stripping of parietal pleura
   D. instillations of nitrogen mustard into the pleural space
   E. systemic chemotherapy
   REF: Ibid.

15. A 32-year-old man presents with persistent pain in the right shoulder for three months. His right pupil is noted to be contracted and the muscles of the thenar eminence are atrophied. A chest film taken two months previously was passed as normal. Which of the following tests is likely to be most helpful?
   A. bronchoscopy
   B. full plate tomography of the lungs
   C. sputum cytology
   D. special radiographic views to show upper right ribs and vertebrae
   E. alkaline phosphatase
   REF: Ibid.
   Crofton, J. and Douglas, A.: *Respiratory Diseases, 2nd Ed.*, J.B. Lippincott, Philadelphia, 1975, p. 511

16. Chemotherapy is likely to be beneficial in lung cancer under which of the following circumstances?
   A. superior vena cava obstruction
   B. pericardial involvement
   C. the histological type of the tumor has been shown to be an adenocarcinoma
   D. fibrinolysin has been demonstrated in the blood
   E. vertebral metastases
   REF: Baum, G.L. (Ed.): *Textbook of Pulmonary Diseases, 2nd Ed.*, Little, Brown and Company, Boston 1974, Chapter 35

17. A 27-year-old woman presents with weakness, edema and darkening of the skin. She has also become slightly hirsute and has put on 24 pounds. Her electrolytes were determined and the following results were obtained: sodium 144 mEq/l, potassium cortisol was 90 g/100 ml and after a diagnostic test with metyrapone, the level was 93 g/100 ml. The probable diagnosis is
    A. bronchial adenoma
    B. thymoma secreting ectopic ACTH
    C. adrenal carcinoma
    D. oat cell carcinoma of the bronchus
    REF: Ibid., Chapter 38

18. A 36-year-old man is seen with a three-month history of nausea, vomiting, abdominal pain, weakness and mental confusion. Physical examination serves only to confirm that the patient is confused, weak and has severe hiccoughs. An electroencephalograph shows diffuse nonspecific changes, while a chest film shows a solid 5 cm circumscribed lesion in the periphery of the lower lobe. Which one of the following tests is most likely to confirm the suspected diagnosis?
    A. serum sodium
    B. alkaline phosphatase
    C. serum calcium
    D. serum magnesium
    E. estimation of 5-hydroxyindoleacetic acid in urine
    F. plasma cortisol level
    REF: Ibid.

19. A 52-year-old man presents with a six week history of depression, lethargy and muscular weakness, and a subnormal temperature. Three days prior to admission he had become confused and semicomatose following drinking several glasses of water. A chest film shows a left hilar mass. His serum calcium is normal. Which of the following laboratory findings might be expected to be present?
A. serum sodium 112 mEq/l
B. serum sodium 152 mEq/l
C. urinary sodium in 24 hours 170 mEq/l
D. simultaneous demonstration of a plasma osmolality of 250 mOsm/kg and a urine osmolality of 650 mOsm/kg
E. total body water 23% of body weight
REF: Ibid.

20. A 50-year-old man presents with pain and swelling in the fingers, wrists, and ankles. He has lost five pounds, and on examination he has clubbing of the fingers and toes, and swelling of the above-mentioned joints. Radiographs of his ankles show subperiosteal new bone formation, and hypertrophic pulmonary osteoarthropathy is diagnosed. Which of the following conditions might he have?
A. tuberculosis
B. pachydermoperiostosis
C. pyogenic lung abscess
D. pulmonary metastases
E. bronchogenic carcinoma
REF: Baum, G.L. (Ed.): *Textbook of Pulmonary Diseases,* 2nd Ed., Little, Brown and company, Boston, 1974, pp. 827-828

21. In the patient mentioned above a bronchogenic carcinoma was seen on chest radiography. Which of the following procedures might cause regression of the osteoarthropathy?
A. resection of the tumor
B. corticosteroids
C. androgens
D. exploratory thoracotomy
E. vagotomy
REF: Ibid., pp. 827-830

22. A 44-year-old woman presents with an obscure anemia. This turns out to be due to pure red cell aplasia. A chest film shows a mass to be present. Where is it likely to be located?
    A. at one of the HeLa
    B. in the posterior mediastinum
    C. in the mid mediastinum
    D. in the anterior mediastinum
    E. in the right paratracheal region
    REF: Ibid., p. 832

23. A 45-year-old man was admitted with a history of Hodgkin's disease diagnosed two years previously. He had been treated initially with melphalan (Alkeran) but is now receiving vincristine and prednisone. He has experienced increasingly more severe chest pain over the past two weeks. In that two-week interval, cavitated nodular lesions have appeared on his chest x-ray. Which of the following assumptions is most likely?
    A. the nodular lesions represent metastatic disease refractory to the present treatment
    B. the nodular lesions represent multiple streptococcal abscesses
    C. the nodular lesions represent a fungal infection
    D. the nodular lesions represent a reaction to drugs used in the therapy of Hodgkin's disease
    REF: Crofton, J. and Douglas, A.: *Respiratory Diseases, 2nd Ed.*, J.B. Lippincott, Philadelphia 1975, Chapter 18

24. Which of the following agents may produce pulmonary emphysema?
    A. bauxite
    B. limestone
    C. isocyanates
    D. vanadium
    E. cadmium
    REF: Morgan, W.K.C. and Seaton, A.: *Occupational Lung Diseases*, W.B. Saunders Company, Philadelphia, 1975, Chapter 16

25. Progressive massive fibrosis may be found in
    A. berylliosis
    B. hematite miners' lung
    C. kaolin lung
    D. asbestosis
    E. graphite lung
    REF: Ibid., p. 129

26. Which of the following statements are true of chronic berylliosis?
    A. sarcoidosis may be distinguished from berylliosis by an analysis of a biopsy specimen for its beryllium content
    B. spontaneous resolution occurs in sarcoidosis but not in berylliosis
    C. hypergammaglobulinemia is more common in sarcoidosis
    D. berylliosis influences tuberculin sensitivity
    E. hilar adenopathy without parenchymal involvement does not occur in berylliosis
    REF: Ibid., Chapter 11

27. Which of the following statements are true of the simple coal workers' pneumoconiosis?
    A. focal emphysema is a common pathologic finding
    B. the most important element in the pathogenesis is silica
    C. the disease is only found in underground coal workers
    D. it rarely produces respiratory impairment in the absence of obstructive airway disease
    E. it predisposes to tuberculosis
    REF: Ibid., Chapter 10

28. A 43-year-old coal miner is referred to a chest clinic because his chest x-ray shows multiple opacities in his lungs. These opacities are peripherally situated. He has no symptoms. Physical examination is within normal limits. His blood count and urinalysis are normal, but his erythrocyte sedimentation rate is elevated to 32 mm in one hour. Which of the following tests or investigations is likely to provide the strongest circumstantial evidence of the correct diagnosis?
    A. an intravenous pyelogram
    B. complement fixation test for histoplasmosis
    C. barium enema
    D. latex fixation test for rheumatoid factor
    E. intermediate PPD skin test
    REF: Ibid.

29. A 40-year-old demolition worker presents with increasing exertional dyspnea of a 12-month duration. He also has a dry cough, though he has never been a smoker. He is seen to be cyanosed and to have finger clubbing. Examination of the chest is normal, apart from a tachypnea and a few fine basilar inspiratory crepitations. However, the chest radiograph shows a reticular appearance in the lung fields and a shaggy appearance to the cardiac border. Calcification is seen on the diaphragmatic pleura. The most likely diagnosis is
    A. silicosis
    B. Shaver's disease
    C. mesothelioma
    D. asbestosis
    E. idiopathic interstitial fibrosis
    REF: Ibid., Chapter 9

30. Which of the following occupations may entail a risk of the development of silicosis?
    A. enameling
    B. abrasive soap manufacturing
    C. silver polishing
    D. corundum smelting
    E. gold mining
    REF: Ibid., Chapter 7

31. Disodium cromoglycate (Intal)
    A. is useful in the management of all types of bronchoconstriction
    B. inhibits the release of bronchoconstrictor substances
    C. reduces the bronchoconstriction
    D. may be given orally or by injection
    E. acts on the alpha-receptors in the bronchial smooth muscle
    REF: Baum, G.L. (Ed.): *Textbook of Pulmonary Diseases,* 2nd Ed., Little, Brown and Company, Boston, 1974, p. 434

32. Which of the following features are characteristic of primary emphysema (pink puffer)?
    A. a small heart and dilated proximal arteries on chest radiograph
    B. severe airway obstruction
    C. slight or no hypoxemia and a normal $PaCO_2$
    D. a clinical course marked by progressive dyspnea and little sputum production
    E. recurrent episodes of cor pulmonale
    REF: Crofton, J. and Douglas, A.: *Respiratory Diseases,* 2nd Ed., J.B. Lippincott, Philadelphia, 1975, p. 338

33. Destruction of alveolar walls is typically found in
    A. compensatory emphysema
    B. focal emphysema of coal workers' pneumoconiosis
    C. panacinar emphysema
    D. senile emphysema
    E. ball-valve obstructive emphysema
    REF: Ibid., p. 332

Pulmonary / 185

34. A 30-year-old man presents with mild dyspnea and a history of mild chronic bronchitis. Examination reveals slight deviation of the trachea to the left, and overinflation and increased resonance to percussion on the right side. Breath sounds are reduced on the right side. Which of the following diagnoses is consistent with these findings?
    A. right upper lobe bullous disease
    B. right Macleod's syndrome
    C. right pleural effusion
    D. collapse of right upper lobe
    E. cavitation of right upper lobe
    REF: Ibid., pp. 348-351

35. In the management of "shock lung" (ARDS), institution of positive end expiratory pressure (PEEP) may result in which of the following complications?
    A. pneumothorax
    B. reduced cardiac output
    C. oxygen toxicity
    D. pneumomediastinum
    E. gastric dilatation
    REF: Baum, G.L. (Ed.): *Textbook of Pulmonary Diseases*, 2nd Ed., Little, Brown and Company, Boston, 1974, Chapter 29

36. A 47-year-old man develops septic shock on his eighth hospital day and becomes apneic. Mechanical ventilation is instituted along with antibiotics, steroids and volume replacement. Eight hours later, the patient demonstrated Trousseau and Chvostek signs. Which of the following conditions may result in this chemical picture?
    A. metabolic acidosis
    B. respiratory alkalosis
    C. hypokalemia
    D. hypocalcemia
    E. hypomagnesemia
    REF: J. Hopkins Med. J. 138:53-61, 1976

37. Which of the following statements are true about lung scans using macroaggregated human albumin?
    A. it is entirely safe
    B. allergic reactions have been reported
    C. large particle size has been implicated as the cause of death in some patients
    D. excessive doses in patients with contracted pulmonary bed have resulted in fatalities
    REF: Br. Heart J. 35:917, 1973

38. Which of the following is the most effective way of reducing the incidence of fat embolism after bone fractures?
    A. heparin
    B. low molecular weight dextran
    C. intravenous corticosteroids
    D. hypertonic glucose administration
    E. phenformin
    REF: Arch. Intern. Med. 133:288, 1974

39. A patient is suspected of having a pulmonary embolism. Which of the following tests would be useful to demonstrate iliac vein thrombosis?
    A. ^{131}I fibrinogen uptake
    B. Doppler ultrasonic test
    C. intratrochanteric phlebography
    D. clinical examination
    E. all of the above
    REF: Crofton J. and Douglas A., *Respiratory Diseases, 2nd Ed.*, J.B. Lippincott, Philadelphia, 1975, p. 492

40. In the surgical patient, tests with ^{125}I labelled fibrinogen have shown that the onset of leg vein thrombosis is most likely to occur
    A. at the time of surgery
    B. before surgery
    C. two days after surgery
    D. five days after surgery
    E. ten days after surgery
    REF: Br. Med. J. 1:603, 1974

41. Which of the following statements are true about amphotericin B?
    A. it precipitates in saline solution
    B. ototoxicity is a common complication with use of this drug
    C. heparin may be infused with this drug to reduce incidence of phlebitis
    D. minimal dose (total) of this drug should be one gram
    E. it should not be used with 5-fluorocytosine because of greatly increased renal toxicity
    REF: Busey, J.F.: Clinical Notes on Respiratory Diseases, Spring 1976, p. 226
    Baum, G.L. (Ed.): *Textbook of Pulmonary Diseases, 2nd Ed.*, Little, Brown and Company, Boston, 1974, p. 233

42. A 47-year-old woman is seen with a six-month history of joint pains. She is diagnosed as having early rheumatoid arthritis and is put on aspirin. She develops a "reaction" to the aspirin. Which of the following effects or lesions are commonly seen in subjects who react to aspirin?
    A. asthma
    B. fleeting infiltrates in the lung
    C. nasal polyps
    D. rash
    E. lymphadenopathy
    REF: Crofton, J. and Douglas, A.: *Respiratory Diseases, 2nd Ed.*, J.B. Lippincott, Philadelphia, 1975, p. 433

43. Complications of an initial attack of acute pancreatitis may include
    A. elevated calcium level
    B. glucose intolerance
    C. elevated serum potassium
    D. elevated glucagon level
    E. pleural effusion
    REF: Ibid., p. 284
    Ann. Intern. Med. 83:778, 1975

44. A 38-year-old man who is being treated with antibiotics for bilateral lower lobe lung abscesses has a brisk hemoptysis. It is estimated that he lost 600 ml over a period of two hours, and shortly after the onset of hemoptysis he experienced marked respiratory distress and became cyanosed. These symptoms gradually improved; however, he continued to bleed. His BP and pulse remained at 120/80 mm Hg and 94 respectively. Shortly after the acute episode, he was cross matched. Which of the following procedures or therapeutic regimens is indicated above?
   A. bronchography
   B. bronchoscopy
   C. start patient on vasopressin
   D. tracheostomy
   E. whole blood transfusion
   REF: Crofton, J. and Douglas, A.: *Respiratory Diseases, 2nd Ed.*, J.B. Lippincott, Philadelphia, 1975, Chapter 42

45. Pneumothorax occurs in the newborn most frequently in association with which of the following conditions?
   A. meconium aspiration
   B. tracheoesophageal fistula
   C. hyaline membrane disease
   D. postmature syndrome
   E. normal newborns
   REF: Br. Med. J. 4:310, 1975

46. Which of the following statements is true about fire-caused inhalation of toxic combustion products?
   A. soot particles may reach the alveoli and cause inflammation because of absorbed irritants
   B. HCl in the gaseous phase reaches the alveolus
   C. mucosal irritation by HCl gas will warn of potential danger
   D. the major danger in polyvinylchloride polymer fires is the production of phosgene
   E. HCl inhalation causes immediate respiratory difficulty
   REF: J.A.M.A. 235:393, 1976 (Jan. 26)

47. Which of the following is the main hazard of the inhalation of methylene chloride (CH_2Cl_2) paint removers?
    A. liver toxicity of CH_2Cl_2
    B. respiratory failure due to CH_2Cl_2
    C. acute noncardiac pulmonary edema due to CH_2Cl_2
    D. carbon monoxide poisoning
    E. reduced pulmonary surfactant production
    REF: J.A.M.A. 235:398, 1976 (Jan. 26)

48. A 14-year-old boy is seen with defects in the membranous bones, diabetes insipidus and a chest x-ray showing reticulonodulation. Microscopically, the lungs might be expected to show which of the following features?
    A. histiocytic cellular infiltration
    B. foamy macrophages
    C. fibroblastic proliferation
    D. plasma cell infiltration
    E. proteinaceous deposits in alveoli
    REF: Crofton, J. and Douglas, A.: *Respiratory Diseases, 2nd Ed.*, J.B. Lippincott, Philadelphia, 1975, p. 620
    Spencer, H.: *Pathology of the Lung, 2nd Ed.*, Pergamon Press, New York, 1968, Chapter 21

49. A 37-year-old white male is referred because of difficulty in staying awake. His height is 5'-10" and his weight is 280 lbs. On examination, the skin appeared somewhat plethoric, chest expansion was normal and no abnormal sounds were detected on auscultation of the chest. Which of the following would be expected findings?
    A. a maximal breathing capacity (maximal voluntary ventilation) of 50% of predicted normal
    B. an arterial oxygen saturation of 95%
    C. expiratory reserve volume (ERV) that is 50% of predicted normal in the recumbent position
    D. an FEV_1/FVC ratio of less than 60% of predicted normal
    REF: Bates, D.V., Macklem, P., and Christie, R.V.: *Respiratory Function in Disease, 2nd Ed.*, W.B. Saunders Company, Philadelphia, 1971, Chapter 16

50. Which of the following illnesses may produce pulmonary cavitation?
    A. Klebsiella pneumonia
    B. coal workers' pneumoconiosis
    C. Wegener's granulomatosis
    D. aspergilloma
    E. pulmonary embolism
    REF: Crofton, J. and Douglas, A.: *Respiratory Diseases, 2nd Ed.*, J.B. Lippincott, Philadelphia, 1975, pp. 137, 475, 497, 517

51. Pulmonary edema may occur in which of the following circumstances?
    A. removal of pleural effusion by thoracentesis
    B. pulmonary alveolar proteinosis
    C. Hamman-Rich syndrome
    D. phosgene inhalation
    E. ozone inhalation
    REF: Ibid., pp. 295, 530, 532

52. An 18-year-old man is transferred to your service after abdominal surgery revealed extensive abdominal lymphosarcoma. He is tachypneic at rest and has dullness to percussion in both hemithoraces. Chest x-ray shows bilateral pleural effusions, hilar adenopathy and mediastinal widening. Initial treatment should include
    A. mediastinoscopy
    B. diuretics
    C. thoracentesis
    D. mediastinal radiation
    E. tracheotomy
    REF: Baum, G.L. (Ed.): *Textbook of Pulmonary Diseases, 2nd Ed.*, Little, Brown and Company, Boston, 1974, p. 811

53. Which of the following statements are true in hypertrophic pulmonary osteoarthropathy?
   A. it is most often associated with carcinoma of the bronchus
   B. it will disappear after removal of a chest tumor
   C. it always indicates bronchogenic carcinoma
   D. section of vagus nerve may abolish it
   E. serum growth hormone is always raised in these patients
   REF: Baum, G.L. (Ed.): *Textbook of Pulmonary Diseases,* *2nd Ed.*, Little, Brown and Company, Boston, 1974, pp. 827-830
   Crofton, J. and Douglas, A.: *Respiratory Diseases, 2nd Ed.*, J.B. Lippincott, Philadelphia, 1975, p. 578

54. A 24-year-old teacher complains of decreased exercise tolerance, arthralgia, and sandy feeling in her eyes. A synovial biopsy showed a single noncaseating granuloma. A further diagnostic test likely to be most productive is
   A. serum protein electrophoresis
   B. rectal mucosa biopsy
   C. conjunctival biopsy
   D. serum calcium
   REF: Ibid., Chapter 28

55. Which of the following statements are true of the diagnosis of pneumococcal pneumonia?
   A. sputum gram stains are diagnostic
   B. sputum culture as often reflects the flora of the nasopharynx as it does the flora of the lower respiratory tract
   C. the quellung reaction identifies pneumococci in sputum or cultures
   D. resistant pneumococci (to penicillin) are seen in five percent of pneumonia caused by pneumococci
   E. sputum culture shows distinctive dimpling of the colonies at 48 hours
   REF: Baum, G.L. (Ed.): *Textbook of Pulmonary Diseases,* *2nd Ed.*, Little, Brown and Company, Boston, 1974, Chapter 7

X: Oncology

DIRECTIONS: For each of the following questions or incomplete statements, **ONE** or **MORE** of the answers or completions given is correct. Select:
    A if only 1, 2 and 3 are correct,
    B if only 1 and 3 are correct,
    C if only 2 and 4 are correct,
    D if only 4 is correct,
    E if all are correct.

1. Stage III or IV, asymptomatic, non-Hodgkin's lymphomas that do **NOT** need to be started on chemotherapy include
   1. histiocytic lymphomas
   2. nodular poorly differentiated lymphocytic lymphomas
   3. nodular mixed lymphocytic lymphomas
   4. nodular lymphocytic well-differentiated lymphomas
   REF: Ann. Intern. Med. 90:10, 1979

2. In breast cancer, combination chemotherapy as opposed to single agent sequential chemotherapy
   1. increases complete remissions
   2. increases total percentage of objective responses
   3. is generally more toxic
   4. increases life expectancy
   REF: Seminars in Oncology 5:417, 1978
   Clinical Research 27:53A, February, 1979

3. Tamoxifen (ICI 46474) in metastatic breast cancer
   1. is useful in estrogen receptor negative tumors
   2. can produce regressions in both pre- and postmenopausal women
   3. is given IV weekly
   4. is an antiestrogen
   REF: Ann. Intern. Med. 87:687, 1977

4. Estrogen receptors in breast cancer are
   1. more commonly positive and to a higher value in postmenopausal women compared to premenopausal women
   2. valuable in predicting response to hormonal manipulation
   3. generally similarly positive or negative in the primary and metastases
   4. usually negative in axillary metastases
   REF: Cancer Research 38:4296, 1978

5. Adjunctive chemotherapy has been demonstrated to increase the "cure" rate in
   1. carcinoma of the colon
   2. melanoma
   3. squamous cell carcinoma of the lung
   4. premenopausal breast cancer
   REF: N. Engl. J. Med. 294:405, 1976

Directions Summarized				
A	B	C	D	E
1, 2, 3 only	1, 3 only	2, 4 only	4 only	All are correct

6. Histiocytic lymphoma
   1. usually involves the bone marrow at presentation
   2. can be cured with multiagent chemotherapy
   3. is usually nodular
   4. has a better prognosis if large, cleaved type

   REF: N. Engl. J. Med. 299:1383, 1978

7. Immunoblastic lymphadenopathy is a recent disease entity characterized by
   1. immunoblastic proliferation in nodes with arborizing small vessels and amorphous eosinophilic material
   2. fever, sweats, weight loss and rash
   3. generalized lymphadenopathy, often with hepatosplenomegaly
   4. poor prognosis

   REF: N. Engl. J. Med. 292:1, 1975

8. *Cis*-diaminodichloroplatinum is a chemotherapeutic agent that
   1. clinically causes nausea and vomiting in the majority of cases
   2. causes renal and liver toxicity
   3. induces hearing loss and bone marrow depression
   4. is eliminated through the lungs

   REF: Ann. Intern. Med. 86:803, 1977

9. Oat cell carcinoma of the lung
   1. is usually centrally located in the chest
   2. frequently involves the bone marrow
   3. responds well to chemotherapy and radiation
   4. should be treated initially with surgery

   REF: Ann. Intern. Med. 88:522, 1977

10. Most surgeons feel that patients with primary malignant melanoma should have dissection of the regional nodes if
    1. the lesion is Clark's level IV
    2. the lesion is nonpigmented
    3. the lesion is greater than 1.5 mm thick, according to Breslow's classification
    4. the patient is anergic
    REF: Cancer 43:883, 1979

11. Nonspecific immunotherapy with BCG in primary malignant melanoma, with no known metastases
    1. increases the cure rate
    2. delays recurrence
    3. is innocuous
    4. can occasionally lead to systemic BCG infection
    REF: N. Engl. J. Med. 294:237, 1976

12. Chemotherapeutic agents that are active in primary brain tumors include
    1. VM-26 (podophyllotoxin)
    2. procarbazine
    3. BCNU (nitrosourea)
    4. fluorouracil
    REF: J. Surg. Oncol. 10:543, 1978

13. Agents that are helpful in reducing the hypercalcemia of malignancy include
    1. mithramycin
    2. oral phosphosoda
    3. calcitonin
    4. Indocin
    REF: Ca. - A Cancer Journal for Clinicians 27:258, 1977

14. Complications of radiation and chemotherapy treatment of Hodgkin's disease include
    1. pericardial effusion
    2. transverse myelitis
    3. acute leukemia
    4. prolonged myelosuppression
    REF: Cancer 43:1234, 1979

	Directions Summarized			
A 1, 2, 3 only	B 1, 3 only	C 2, 4 only	D 4 only	E All are correct

15. Chemotherapy agents that lead to renal injury include
    1. methyl CCNU
    2. hydrea
    3. streptozotocin
    4. procarbazine
    REF: N. Engl. J. Med. 300:1200, 1979

16. Metastatic carcinoma of the kidney can regress when treated with
    1. progestational agents
    2. CCNU (vinblastine)
    3. specific and nonspecific immunotherapy
    4. fluorouracil
    REF: Proc. Am. Soc. Clin. Onc. 19:316, 1978; 20:348, 1979

17. A recently described combination chemotherapy for disseminated testicular carcinomas consisting of *cis*-diaminodichloroplatinum, bleomycin and vinblastine
    1. is not active in seminomas
    2. produces a greater than 75% objective response
    3. is nontoxic
    4. effects probable cures
    REF: Ann. Intern. Med. 87:293, 1977

18. Chemicals associated with the development of human liver tumors include
    1. vinyl chloride
    2. androgens
    3. oral contraceptives
    4. prednisone
    REF: Int. J. Gynec. Obstet. 15:137, 1977
        N. Engl. J. Med. 292:17, 1975

DIRECTIONS: Each of the questions or incomplete statements below is followed by five suggestions or completions. Select the **one** that is **BEST** in each case.

19. Preoperative radiation appears to be of value in decreasing local recurrence in
    A. biliary carcinoma
    B. Hodgkin's disease
    C. carcinoma of the rectum
    D. adrenal carcinoma
    E. none of the above
    REF: Cancer 35:1597, 1975

20. An inherited translocation between chromosomes 3 and 8 is associated with the development of
    A. carcinoma of the adrenal
    B. carcinoma of the colon
    C. carcinoma of the kidney
    D. myelomonocytic leukemia
    E. chronic lymphatic leukemia
    REF: N. Engl. J. Med. 301:592, 1979

21. A chemotherapeutic agent of use in ovarian carcinoma is
    A. 6-mercaptopurine
    B. DTIC
    C. hydrea
    D. hexamethylmelamine
    E. OP'DDD
    REF: N. Engl. J. Med. 299:1261, 1978

22. An agent useful in the treatment of the malignant carcinoid syndrome is
    A. DTIC
    B. OP'DDD
    C. BCG
    D. calcitonin
    E. Indocin
    REF: Ca. Treatment Reports 61:101, 1977

Directions Summarized				
A	B	C	D	E
1, 2, 3 only	1, 3 only	2, 4 only	4 only	All are correct

23. Ovarian carcinomas are frequently understaged at initial staging surgery because of
    A. inadequate preoperative work-up
    B. failure to examine and biopsy the liver
    C. failure to adequately explore the diaphragm surfaces
    D. failure to take adequate biopsies of iliac nodes
    E. none of the above
    REF: Cancer 39:967, 1977

24. A promising chemotherapy combination in head and neck tumors is
    A. 6-mercaptopurine and BCG
    B. fluorouracil and L-asparaginase
    C. camptothecin and mithramycin
    D. OP'DDD and prednisone
    E. *cis*-diaminodichloroplatinum, methotrexate and bleomycin
    REF: Proc. Am. Soc. Clin. Onc. 20:384, 1979

25. In colorectal carcinoma a more effective combination of agents than fluorouracil alone is
    A. FU and hydrea
    B. FU and methyl CCNU
    C. methyl CCNU and dacarbazine
    D. FU + methyl CCNU + dacarbazine + vincristine
    E. none of the above
    REF: Proc. Am. Soc. Clin. Onc. 19:384, 1978.

Answers and Comments

The authors have made every effort to thoroughly verify the following answers to the questions which appear on the preceding pages. However, as in any text, some inaccuracies and ambiguities may occur; therefore, if in doubt, please consult your references.

THE PUBLISHER

among "aluminum-only" antacids...

The better alternative

AlternaGEL™ ANTACID (aluminum hydroxide, Stuart)

With preferred flavor,* higher potency and lower sodium content than the leading aluminum hydroxide antacid.

For cases where magnesium-containing antacids are undesirable:

☐ Patients with renal insufficiency.
☐ Patients with GI complications resulting from steroid or other drug therapy.
☐ Patients experiencing laxation which sometimes occurs with continuing high doses of magnesium or combination antacid regimens.

*Independent research data, available on request.

STUART PHARMACEUTICALS | Division of ICI Americas Inc. | Wilmington, DE 19897

I: Cardiology
Answers and Comments

1. C. Isolated rupture of chordae tendineae is responsible for 19% of cases of mitral regurgitation, whereas rheumatic mitral regurgitation is still responsible for 39% of cases.

2. D. The major indication for coronary artery bypass has been and continues to be relief of chronic, disabling angina pectoris.

3. C. All of the answers are found as antecedents to newly acquired LBBB, but hypertension is found in 73% vs 38% in controls ($p < 0.01$).

4. D. Bronchospasm induced by β-blockers can be reversed by aminophylline or isoproterenol.

5. C. The hypotensive potential of prazosin is a result of the specificity for postsynaptic α-receptor blockade.

6. E. Evaluation of its therapy has been clouded by the multiple definitions.

7. C. Without the degree of symptomatic relief afforded by coronary artery bypass surgery, it would not be acceptable to continue a procedure with a 10% to 15% perioperative rate of myocardial infarction.

8. B. Arrhythmias causing severe symptoms require therapy.

9. A. Radionuclide assessment of regional myocardial perfusion is noninvasive and safe.

10. D. None of these tracers possess ideal physical and biologic properties.

Tastemaster

MYLANTA® LIQUID/TABLETS
(aluminum and magnesium hydroxides with simethicone)

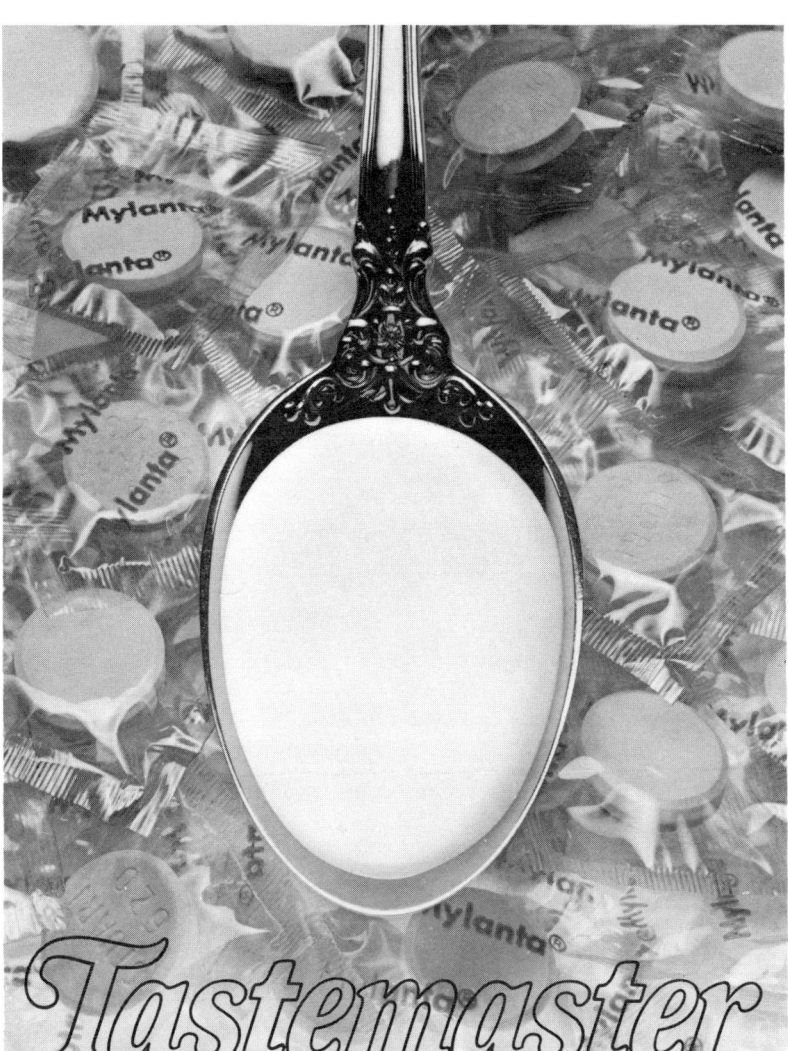

LOW SODIUM ANTACID/ANTIFLATULENT
FOR ROUTINE HYPERACIDITY.
GREAT TASTE FOR GREATER COMPLIANCE.

STUART PHARMACEUTICALS
Division of ICI Americas Inc.
Wilmington, Delaware 19897

Copyright © 1979 ICI Americas Inc.

11. A. Other chambers are not normally visualized owing to thinner walls and lower blood supply.

12. B. There are physiologic areas of decreased perfusion in the normal myocardium.

13. C. Drugs should be used as an adjunct to diet.

14. B. The optimal values of serum cholesterol range from 170–240 mg/dl.

15. D. Bile acid–binding resins may decrease serum cholesterol by up to 50%.

16. B. Transiently decreased arterial pressure lowers the ventricular afterload, which permits greater shortening of muscle fibers.

17. A. Coronary blood flow is a physiologic determinant of myocardial oxygen supply.

18. C. Usual age range is 50 ± 12 years.

19. D. Congestive heart failure occurs in 54% of cases.

20. B. A low pH *may* produce an effect on action potential duration.

21. C. Dyspnea occurs in 85% of cases of constrictive pericarditis.

22. B. Neck veins are distended in 95% of patients with constrictive pericarditis.

23. C. The surgical mortality for pericardiectomy in pericardial constriction is low (5%–10%).

24. D. Blood cultures are positive in approximately 85% of patients with infective endocarditis.

25. B. More than six blood cultures are rarely necessary.

MYLANTA-II
(aluminum and magnesium hydroxides with simethicone)

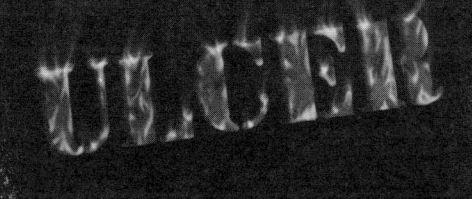

HIGH-POTENCY ANTACID PLUS ANTIFLATULENT
SAFE • EFFECTIVE • PREDICTABLE
AND
LOWEST IN SODIUM

STUART PHARMACEUTICALS | Division of ICI Americas Inc. | Wilmington, DE 19897

26. B. The presence of rheumatoid factor correlates with active disease, and titers fall rapidly with adequate therapy.

27. D. Mouth flora have an ability not found in other organisms to adhere to heart valves.

28. C. Tachycardia leads to increased myocardial oxygen demand.

29. D. Serious ventricular arrhythmia at rest, refractory to therapy, is another absolute contraindication to exercise testing.

30. A. Other absolute indications include declining blood pressure or heart rate, ventricular tachycardia, ataxia, and vertigo.

31. B. Prazosin is taken up rapidly by various tissues.

32. D. After the first dose of prazosin, some patients develop severe orthostatic hypotension, lightheadedness, dizziness, weakness, or palpitations.

33. B. Total plasma creatine kinase lacks specificity for the diagnosis of acute myocardial infarction with a false-positive incidence of about 15%.

34. C. MB creatine kinase is confined virtually exclusively to myocardial cells.

35. C. The concentration of creatine kinase in muscle is 3200 ± 200 IU/gm.

36. A. For survival of a patient in shock following acute myocardial infarction systolic pressure must be at least 80–90 mm Hg for adequate coronary artery perfusion.

37. C. If there is clinical evidence of pulmonary congestion, generally the "wedge" pressure will exceed 18 mm Hg.

38. C. Chronic, low-grade magnesium deficiency may be more common than is thought.

As the gas goes...

so goes the painful gas distress

Mylicon-80 provides prompt and effective antiflatulent activity.

Alters surface tension of the foam which entraps G.I. gas . . . causing the bubbles to coalesce.

Gas is then liberated for easier expulsion...by belching or by passing flatus.

MYLICON®-80 HIGH-CAPACITY ANTIFLATULENT

(simethicone 80 mg.) **STUART PHARMACEUTICALS** | Division of ICI Americas Inc. | Wilmington, DE 19897

39. D. Calcium has 60,000 mEq/70 kg compared with 2000 mEq/70 kg for magnesium.

40. B. Clearance of amylase is reduced.

41. D. This avoids excessive arterial vasoconstriction.

42. C. The high incidence of mitral valve prolapse detected by echocardiography may reflect problems with technique.

43. C. Careful attention to technique, especially with regard to proper position of the transducer and angulation of the beam, is essential.

44. B. A careful history is required if pacemaker malfunction is suspected.

45. D. All grafts develop some morphologic changes with varying functional significance.

46. A. A 90° angle of anastomosis of the vein to aorta is optimal.

47. B. A diastolic murmur of aortic insufficiency also occurs in 58% of patients.

48. D. The presenting symptoms of discrete subaortic stenosis are similar to those of aortic valve stenosis.

49. C. Seventy-five percent of patients have acquired valvular heart disease associated with discrete subaortic stenosis.

50. D. The severity of the rhythm disturbance is not directly related to the severity of subvalve obstruction.

51. C. Less than 320 mg/day is rarely effective, and larger doses are required for maximal benefit.

52. B. It is extremely unusual to use temporary pacing for termination of tachycardias other than atrial flutter.

NEW SODIUM-FREE FORMULATION!

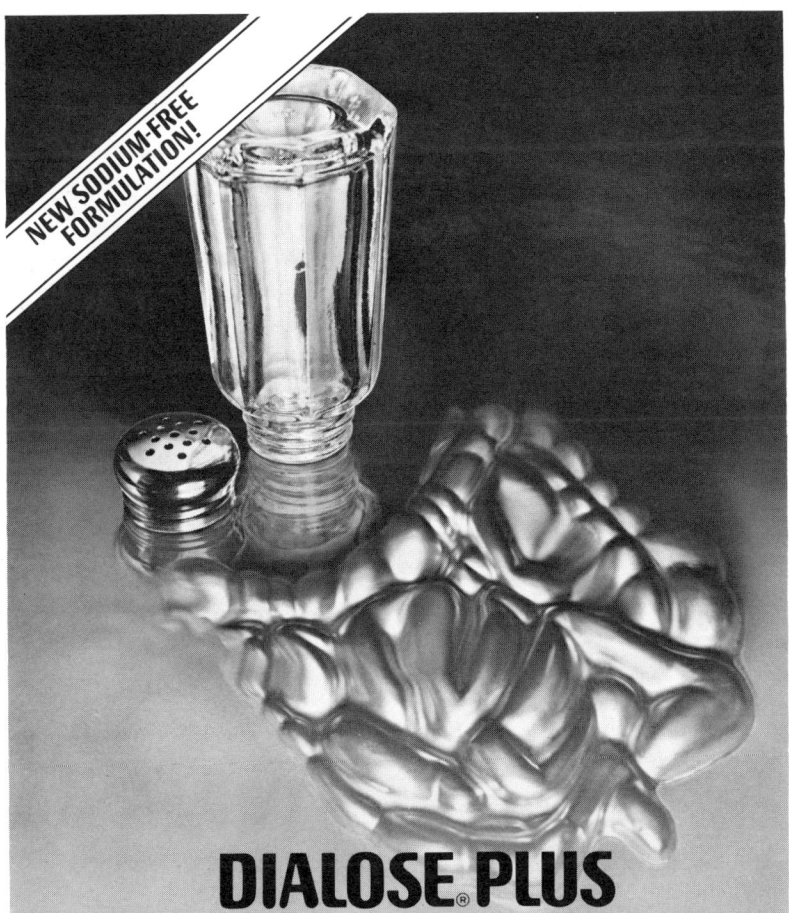

DIALOSE® PLUS
(dioctyl potassium sulfosuccinate, 100 mg.; plus casanthranol, 30 mg.)

An important clinical consideration in treating constipation with a stool softener is not only the selected agent's effectiveness, but also whether or not it contains sodium.

For effectiveness DIALOSE® PLUS contains dioctyl potassium sulfosuccinate, a superior wetting agent that lowers surface tension to soften hard, dry stools. The second component, casanthranol, is a peristaltic activator that increases motor activity of the large intestine, for additional help in elimination.

DIALOSE®PLUS contains no sodium. This means your patients' sodium intake won't be increased when you recommend DIALOSE®PLUS. So for all of your appropriate patients with constipation, make the effective sodium-free move... to DIALOSE®PLUS.

Effective sodium-free move against constipation

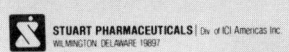

STUART PHARMACEUTICALS | Div of ICI Americas Inc.
WILMINGTON, DELAWARE 19897

53. C. In such patients, atrial fibrillation can be followed by life-threatening high ventricular rates.

54. C. The frequency of "variant" angina depends upon the care with which it is looked for.

55. A. Distinguishing between primary and secondary causes should provide a basis for a rational therapeutic approach to patients with angina at rest.

56. A. Rupture of the papillary muscle usually occurs during the first acute myocardial infarction and the myocardium around the mitral annulus is not damaged.

57. D. Arrhythmias and cardiac failure should be treated based upon their severity.

58. B. It is difficult to predict accurately Type A or Type B behavior, but studies have shown no difference between types for mean resting heart rate and blood pressure, but lability is greater in Type A individuals.

59. E. On the basis of a prospective randomized study interim report, all four choices were statistically significant.

60. C. Patients at risk for infarct expansion are predominantly those with large anterior or anteroseptal infarcts with the major risk period occurring during the first 14 days postinfarct.

61. A. Since the degree of left ventricular dysfunction is a major determinant of morbidity and mortality after acute myocardial infarction, radionuclide assessment can now be used as a noninvasive technique for evaluating biventricular performance.

62. A. Corticosteroids are more effective than aspirin or indomethacin in the treatment of acute pericarditis, but there is no evidence that their use leads to a better outcome.

63. B. The daily dosage ranges between 80 and 480 mg depending on the individual patient's requirements.

Relief...

KASOF®
(dioctyl potassium sulfosuccinate, 240 mg.)

effective stool softener

■ **effective softening action—**
softens hard, dry stools to alleviate painful straining.

■ **sodium-free—**
unique potassium formulation, without the problems associated with sodium intake.

■ **simple one-a-day dosage**

CANDIDATES—the severely constipated, including patients with hemorrhoids and anal fissures.

KASOF...relief with a single daily dose.

STUART PHARMACEUTICALS | Div. of ICI Americas Inc.
WILMINGTON, DELAWARE 19897

64. C. β-blockers do not cause exercise-induced or postural hypotension, patient tolerance is excellent, sedative and CNS side effects are uncommon, and patient compliance is good.

65. A. Almost any viral infection may be accompanied by clinical evidence of altered cardiac function.

66. E. The clinical presentation of viral myocarditis shows wide variations, ranging from total absence of clinical manifestations to sudden unexpected death.

67. B. There are no effective antibiotics for the majority of viruses, and specific therapy for viral diseases is not yet available.

68. D. It is not entirely certain that coronary artery bypass surgery will result in a better prognosis except in significant obstruction of the left main coronary artery.

69. A. The key element is an electrophysiologic derangement that is largely the result of chronic ischemic heart disease.

70. B. A series of useful physiologic events result from treatment of congestive heart failure with vasodilating drugs.

71. A. Nitroglycerin's predominant site of action is the vein.

72. A. The transmural diastolic pressure gradient is a physiologic determinant of myocardial oxygen supply.

73. E. Maximum heart rate may also show no change.

74. B. Other conditions simulated are collagen vascular disease, mitral stenosis, and idiopathic paroxysmal atrial fibrillation.

75. A. Rapid ventricular tachycardia and potassium-losing diuretics also promote potassium loss and arrhythmias.

76. E. Glucose-insulin also decreases myocardial potassium loss.

77. E. The underlying disease in the host may be a factor also.

COMPARISON TASTE TEST:

EFFERSYLLIUM FINISHES...

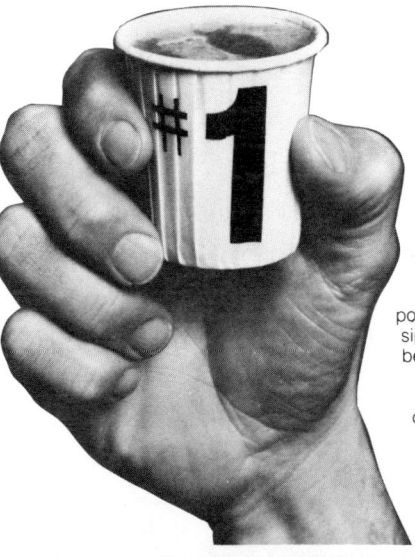

It wasn't surprising. The delicious lemon-lime flavor of Effersyllium appeals to even the most discriminating taste—makes it so much more pleasant to take a bulk laxative. And that's essentially why Effersyllium won out in a nationwide taste test with bulk laxative users.*

Respondents, randomly selected at shopping malls, were asked to taste in sequence equal amounts of two unidentifiable bulk laxatives from identical cups. The Effersyllium and plain Metamucil that were offered for the taste test had already been mixed with cool tap water out of view of the respondents. Moreover, order of presentation was rotated to prevent any position bias. Each taster sipped water before and between tasting the bulk laxatives to clear the palate. When they had completed tasting both products, they were asked, "Now that you have tasted both samples, which taste did you prefer?"

EFFERSYLLIUM® A NAME WORTH REMEMBERING

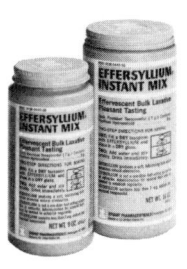

2 out of 3
bulk laxative users preferred the pleasant lemon-lime taste of Effersyllium over Metamucil

STUART PHARMACEUTICALS | Div of ICI Americas Inc.
WILMINGTON, DELAWARE 19897

*Data on file: Stuart Pharmaceuticals

78. A. Most cases of *S. viridans* bacterial endocarditis are responsive to one million units of penicillin IV *q2h* for four weeks.

79. B. Nitroglycerin also maintains cardiac index, heart rate, and stroke volume.

80. A. Blood flow is redistributed from epicardium to endocardium.

81. C. This is a distal tubule potassium-sparing diuretic.

82. C. Its primary effect is inhibiting active chloride transport in the thick ascending portion of the loop of Henle.

83. B. These are distal tubule potassium-wasting diuretics.

84. B. Exercise induced ST-segment elevation is caused by areas of abnormal myocardial wall motion due to a previous myocardial infarction.

85. C. Prazosin is a unique vasodilator in that it does not produce a reflex tachycardia and an increase in renin release.

86. B. These drugs are usually used in the hospital setting.

87. E. Not every patient with hypertension should have treatment started with reserpine or a diuretic.

88. B. Underperfusion and pulmonary congestion must be treated promptly.

89. D. There is no alteration in left ventricular volume produced by propranolol and nitrates in combination.

90. C. Carbon monoxide decreases blood oxygen content and depresses left ventricular function.

91. A. The effects of physical conditioning are additive to those of drugs.

Give them the
COMPLETE
HEMATINIC

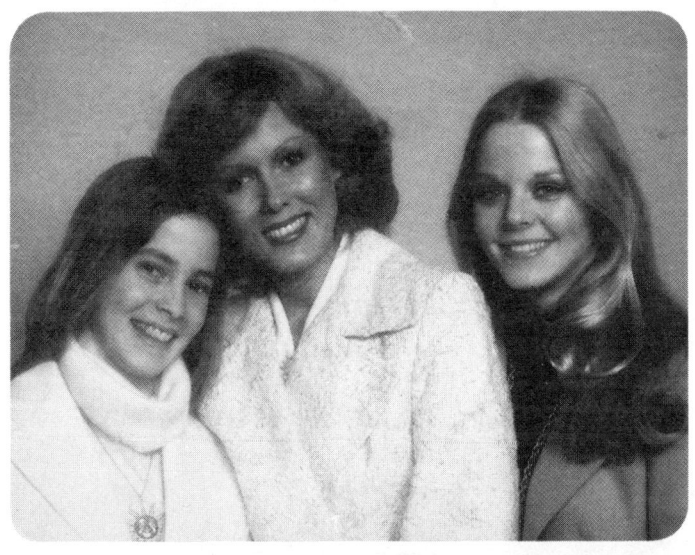

STUARTINIC®

One tablet daily provides:

- *100 mg. elemental iron* (from 300 mg. ferrous fumarate)...as an effective prophylactic measure against anemia
- *B-complex supplementation*...to compensate for possible deficiencies of diet
- *An economical combination* of both the above

STUART PHARMACEUTICALS
Division of ICI Americas Inc.
Wilmington, Delaware 19897

216 / Answers and Comments

92. A. A peaked T wave and widened QRS are seen in moderate magnesium deficiency.

93. E. Bacteremia is rarely complicated by shock in adults under age 40.

94. C. Right ventricular volume overload produces abnormal ventricular septal motion on M-mode echocardiography.

95. E. The chest x-ray is extremely useful in determining the cause of pacemaker malfunction.

96. E. Each factor may vary independently of the other.

97. C. Endothelial and intimal damage may also cause intimal fibrous proliferation.

98. C. The average surgical mortality is 14% in the treatment of hypertrophic obstructive cardiomyopathy.

99. E. Tachycardias can be terminated with the use of appropriately timed electrical stimuli.

100. A. The direction of ST-segment changes corresponds to the extent and distribution of the ischemia.

IRON EFFICIENCY

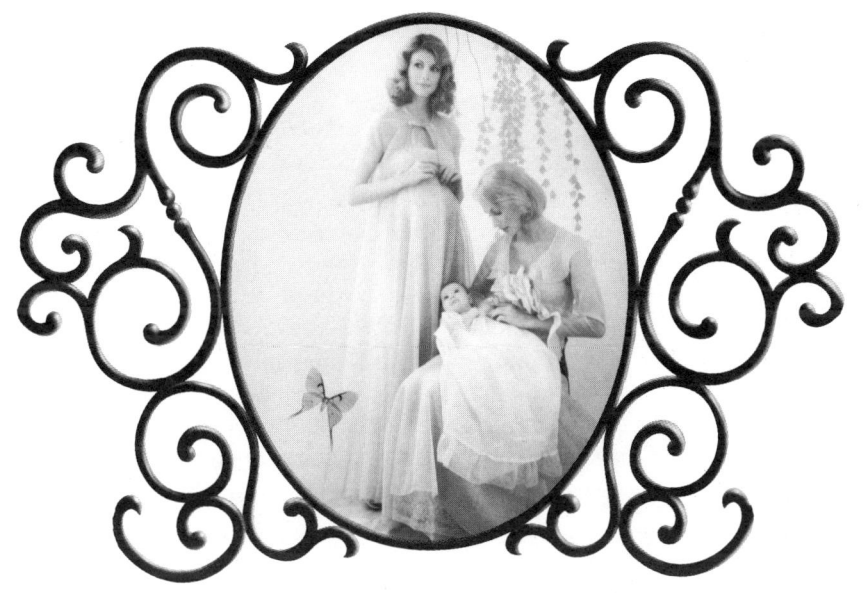

FERANCEE-HP

High potency hematinic for iron deficiency in the perinatal period

Each tablet contains: 110 mg. iron (from 330 mg. ferrous fumarate); 600 mg. vitamin C.

STUART PHARMACEUTICALS
Division of ICI Americas Inc.
Wilmington, DE 19897

II: Hematology
Answers and Comments

1. A. The diffuse lymphocytic lymphomas are somewhat less benign than the nodular variety, although individual cases may well follow a benign and protracted course.

2. D. The median survival of this type is 9.2 years.

3. D. See previous answer.

4. A. Heterophil antibody titers of 1:56 or higher are usually present in untreated serum, and the titers should be 1:28 or higher after the serum has been absorbed with guinea pig kidney.

5. E. Abundance of myeloblasts, 10% or more of the circulating granulocytes, and lysozymuria are other signs of poor prognosis.

6. C. Consumption of fibrinogen and platelets and increased levels of fibrin split products ensue. There is some controversy as to whether DIC or primary fibrinolysis accounts for the hypofibrinogenemia.

7. C. A small number of patients with ALL have T-lymphoblastic leukemia, which is an aggressive disease with poor prognosis.

8. D. About one-third of patients with blastic transformation of chronic granulocytic leukemia are positive for TdT.

9. B. Self-explanatory.

10. E. These basically are the constituents of the MOPP protocol for Hodgkin's disease. Bleomycin, nitrosourea, and anthracycline derivatives are other drugs of value.

11. B. The enzymatic transformation of arachidonic acid to cyclic endoperoxides is inhibited by aspirin or indomethacin.

12. C. The mechanism of platelet destruction in TTP is unknown. Excessive deposition of platelets in cerebral and renal vessels may be responsible for thrombocytopenia in TTP.

13. D. In hemophilia A, by contrast, only the coagulant components of Factor VIII are decreased or absent.

14. C. The other choices listed occur in reactive or secondary thrombocytosis. Autonomous thrombocythemia may occur in patients with polycythemia vera and may precede the appearance of erythrocytosis.

15. D. In one series, 80% of severely affected children were found to have had some impairment of function in the knee joint by the age of 10 years.

16. C. About 10% of patients with hemophilia A develop objective evidence of intracranial hemorrhage.

17. D. There is recent evidence that TTP responds to plasma.

18. B. The effect of heparin is dissipated within six hours.

19. A. Fibrinogen is typically decreased in DIC.

20. A. In one large study, 21 of 512 patients bled excessively after bypass surgery. A bleeding site was found in 13 of these 21 patients. Coagulation studies were normal in all 13 patients.

21. C. The workup of an adult with iron deficiency should never be delayed on the assumption that the anemia is a result of poor diet. Chronic blood loss should always be looked for.

22. C. The presense of an antibody in a patient's serum indicates sensitization by foreign RBC antigens via prior blood transfusion or pregnancy with transplacental exchange of incompatible fetal RBC.

Increasing Sorbitrate to 20mg. q.i.d. could mean improved angina* protection.

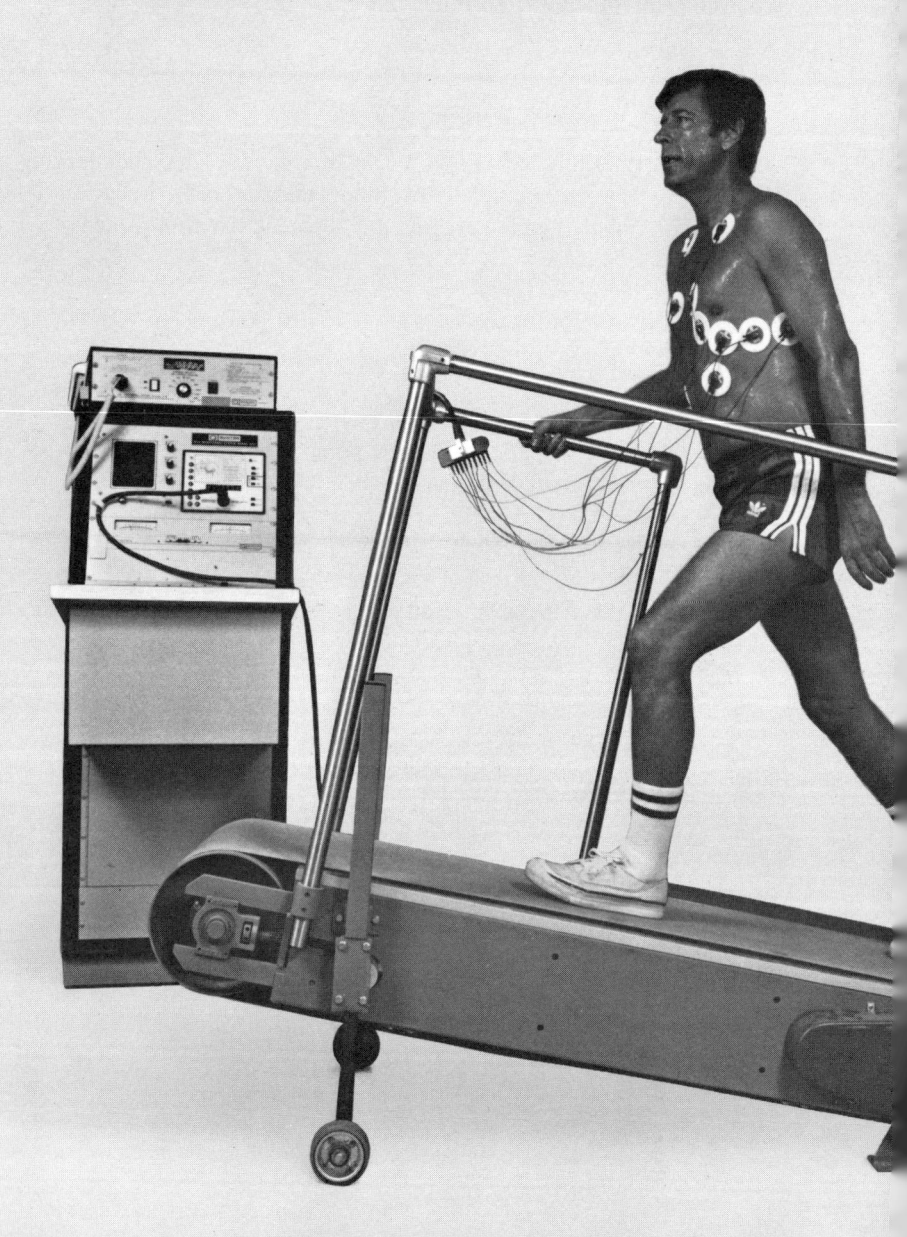

According to recent studies,

higher doses of isosorbide dinitrate significantly improved exercise capacity during standard stress testing.[1-3] Sustained control of angina was also achieved in patients receiving increased doses of isosorbide dinitrate and subsequently stress challenged.[1-3] Headaches, which may occur at initiation of therapy, are usually transient and disappear within two weeks. [2,4,5]

SORBITRATE®
ORAL 20 mg, TABLETS
(ISOSORBIDE DINITRATE)

References: 1. Danahy DT. et al: Sustained hemodynamic and antianginal effect of high-dose oral isosorbide dinitrate. Circulation 55:381-387, February 1977. 2. Danahy DT, Aronow WS: Hemodynamics and antianginal effects of high-dose oral isosorbide dinitrate after chronic use. Circulation 56:205-212, August 1977. 3. Glancy DL, et al: Effect of swallowed isosorbide dinitrate on blood pressure, heart rate and exercise capacity in patients with coronary artery disease. Am J Med 62:39-46, January 1977. 4. Shane SJ: Correspondence; Oral nitrates in angina. Can Med Assoc J 113:360-361, September 6, 1975. 5. Shane SJ: High-dose oral isosorbide dinitrate and ischemic heart pain. Canadian Family Physician 19:61-65, November 1973.

*This drug has been evaluated as possibly effective for this indication. See full prescribing information and references on last page.

STUART PHARMACEUTICALS | Div. of ICI Americas Inc.
Wilmington, DE 19897

SORBITRATE® ISOSORBIDE DINITRATE

DESCRIPTION: Dosage Forms and Strengths

FORMS	STRENGTHS	DESCRIPTION	PACKAGING
CHEWABLE Tablets	5 mg.	Green, round, scored tablets embossed front "STUART", reverse "810"	Bottles of 100 and 500; and Unit Dose package of 100
	10 mg.	Yellow, round, scored tablets embossed front "STUART", reverse "815"	Bottles of 100 and Unit Dose packages of 100
ORAL Tablets	5 mg.	Green, oval-shaped tablets embossed front "STUART", reverse "770"	Bottles of 100 and 500; and Unit Dose packages of 100
	10 mg.	Yellow, oval-shaped tablets embossed front "STUART", reverse "780"	Bottles of 100 and 500; and Unit Dose packages of 100
	20 mg.	Blue, oval-shaped tablets embossed front "STUART", reverse "820"	Bottles of 100 and Unit Dose packages of 100
SA Tablets (Sustained Action)	40 mg.	Yellow, round tablets embossed front "STUART", reverse "880"	Bottles of 100 and Unit Dose packages of 100
SUBLINGUAL Tablets	2.5 mg	Round, white tablets	Bottles of 100 and 500; and Unit Dose packages of 100
	5 mg.	Round, pink tablets	Bottles of 100 and 500; and Unit Dose packages of 100

DESCRIPTION: Chemistry
SORBITRATE® (isosorbide dinitrate) is an organic nitrate that is designated chemically as 1,4:3,6-dianhydrosorbitol-2,5-dinitrate.

MODE OF ACTION: The mechanism of action of SORBITRATE (isosorbide dinitrate) in the relief of angina pectoris is unknown at this time, although the basic pharmacologic action is to relax smooth muscle.

Since therapy at the present time is essentially empirical, clinical improvement is generally measured by a decrease in the severity of the symptoms of angina pectoris and the need for medication. Specifically, SORBITRATE reduces in number and severity the incidence of angina pectoris attacks, with concomitant reduction in nitroglycerin intake.

In the evaluation of isosorbide dinitrate in angina pectoris, clinical improvement has been customarily measured subjectively. Individual patterns of angina pectoris differ widely as does the symptomatic response to antianginal agents. In conjunction with the total management of patients with angina pectoris, isosorbide dinitrate has been generally accepted as safe and widely regarded as useful.

INDICATIONS: Based on a review of this drug by the National Academy of Sciences—National Research Council and/or other information. FDA has classified the indications as follows:

"Probably" effective: Sublingual and chewable dosage forms of SORBITRATE are indicated for the treatment of acute anginal attacks and for prophylaxis in situations likely to provoke such attacks.

"Possibly" effective: Oral dosage forms of SORBITRATE are indicated for the relief of angina pectoris (pain of coronary artery disease). They are not intended to abort the acute anginal episode, but they are widely regarded as useful in the prophylactic treatment of angina pectoris.

Final classification of the less-than-effective indications requires further investigation.

CONTRAINDICATIONS: A history of sensitivity to the drug.
WARNINGS: Data supporting the use of nitrates during the early days of the acute phase of myocardial infarction (the period during which clinical and laboratory findings are unstable) are insufficient to establish safety.
PRECAUTIONS: Tolerance to this drug and cross tolerance to other nitrites and nitrates may occur. All SORBITRATE (isosorbide dinitrate) forms (except Sublinguals and 20 mg. Oral) contain FD&C Yellow No. 5 (tartrazine) which may cause allergic-type reactions (including bronchial asthma) in certain susceptible individuals. Although the overall incidence of FD&C Yellow No. 5 (tartrazine) sensitivity in the general population is low, it is frequently seen in patients who also have aspirin hypersensitivity.

ADVERSE REACTIONS: Headache is the most common adverse reaction and may be severe and persistent. Lowering the dose and use of analgesics will help control the headaches which usually diminish or disappear as therapy is continued. Cutaneous vasodilation with flushing may occur. Transient episodes of dizziness and weakness, as well as other signs of cerebral ischemia associated with postural hypotension, may occasionally develop. This drug can act as a physiological antagonist to norepinephrine, acetylcholine, histamine, and many other agents. An occasional individual exhibits marked sensitivity to the hypotensive effects of nitrates and severe responses (nausea, vomiting, weakness, restlessness, pallor, perspiration, and collapse) can occur even with the usual therapeutic dose. Alcohol may enhance this effect. Drug rash and/or exfoliative dermatitis may occasionally occur.

DOSAGE AND ADMINISTRATION:
Route: Dosage Forms, chewable, sublingual, sustained action, and oral tablets.
Initiating Therapy: In starting patients on SORBITRATE it is necessary to adjust the dosage until the smallest effective dose is determined. This is of particular importance in employing chewable tablets. Occasionally, severe hypotensive responses may occur with this dosage form, even with doses as low as 5 mg.
Individual Dose: 2.5 to 10 mg. is the range commonly used although doses up to 30 mg. have frequently been employed. The oral and chewable tablets are scored for more accurate dosage adjustment when necessary. The usual dose for sustained action tablets is one 40 mg. tablet.
Dosage Schedule: Smallest effective dose necessary for the prevention and treatment of pain of an anginal attack. CHEWABLE SORBITRATE and SORBITRATE Sublingual may be taken P.R.N. for prompt relief of anginal pain, or at 4 to 6 hour intervals. SORBITRATE Oral may be taken 3 to 4 times daily SORBITRATE SA sustained action oral tablets may be taken at 12 hour intervals. Although the onset of effect and the duration of effect of coronary nitrates may be quite variable, following are the generally reported ranges of these values for SORBITRATE.
Onset of Effect:
  Chewable and Sublingual: 2 to 5 minutes
  Oral and Sustained Action: 15 to 30 minutes
Duration of Effect:
  Chewable and Sublingual: 1 to 2 hours
  Oral: Estimated to be 4 to 6 hours
  Sustained Action: Estimated to be up to 12 hours at a continuous controlled rate

It is recommended that the oral dosage be taken on an empty stomach. If vascular headaches cannot be effectively controlled by ordinary measures, dosages may be taken with meals to minimize this side effect.

STUART PHARMACEUTICALS | Div. of ICI Americas Inc.
WILMINGTON, DELAWARE 19897

Answers and Comments / 223

23. D. Typically, in HS, the osmotic fragility of RBC is increased (or the osmotic resistance is decreased) especially after 24 hours incubation at 37°C.

24. D. The blood volume is increased in both disorders.

25. E. The mating of AS x SC results in: AS, AC, SS, SC with 25% probability for each combination.

26. D. Thymectomy may produce a remission or may render drug therapy more successful.

27. C. In pernicious anemia it is not known why the intrinsic factor is not secreted. It is presumed to be a result of autoimmunity.

28. E. New methods of administration of desferrioxamine are promising. Splenectomy decreases the transfusion requirement.

29. C. All other listed items concerning pyruvate kinase deficiency are true.

30. B. Autoimmune hemolytic anemia is the second most common anemia in SLE and affects about 10% of patients.

31. B. Anti-I antibody may also appear as an autoimmune antibody. Anti-I may be found following infectious mononucleosis.

32. C. Venography is an invasive technique that is usually omitted from the initial evaluation because of the associated discomfort. It provides, however, the most definitive information regarding the patency of veins.

33. A. Aplastic crisis in sickle cell anemia causes reticulocytopenia.

34. E. More extensive dental surgery should be carried out after replacement therapy with Factor VIII.

35. E. Other causes include malignant hypertension preeclampsia, disseminated carcinoma, and other collagen vascular diseases.

36. D. Pyroglobulins irreversibly gel at 56°C, whereas Bence Jones proteins precipitate when heated to 56°C, dissolve when heated to boiling and reprecipitate with cooling.

37. C. Other agents such as 6-mercaptopurine or 6-thioguanine are sometimes used in combination with one or both of these drugs.

38. A. Rifampin, like barbiturates and glutethimide, may interfere with the effects of coumarin owing to acceleration of coumarin metabolism.

39. C. The M-component disorders together with 1 and 3 are B-cell disorders.

40. E. The role of splenectomy in aplastic anemia is controversial.

III: Neurology
Answers and Comments

1. B. In a series of patients with Paget's disease, 37 out of 49 had VIII nerve involvement.

2. A. Unilateral frontal headaches were second most common.

3. E. Occlusive extracranial disease occurred in less than 10%.

4. A. Pure hemiparesis or hemiplegia was most consistent. Aphasia, when present, was transient.

5. E. No statistically significant differences were noted in seizure control or acute side effects.

6. A. Memory disorders are early focal signs preceding more widespread intellectual deterioration.

7. B. If mild cases are included, the estimate rises to 11%.

8. B. A 2/1,000 estimated prevalence has been proposed.

9. A. Memory loss occurred in all, disorientation in 80%, agitation in 70%.

10. C. Brainstem emboli were the most common complication in this series.

11. E. All have been reported by several reviewers.

12. B. There is abnormal skin pigmentation and probably abnormal fatty acid degradation.

13. **E.** It may also have features of cerebellar degeneration.

14. **C.** Dopamine hypersensitivity was noted only in patients with Shy-Drager syndrome.

15. **D.** It remains unclear how blood pressure elevation produces headaches.

16. **B.** As more persons live to older age, a greater number seem to develop hypertensive encephalopathy, even though the overall incidence seems to be declining.

17. **A.** All are true, except that the prevalence (2%–3% in general autopsy series) has remained unchanged.

18. **D.** Neurologic complications occur in less than 5% with conventional doses, are mainly cerebellar in type, and relate to each individual dose more than to the total dose.

19. **B.** They usually don't respond to ethosuximide ("petit mal" drug), and at times require temporal lobectomy for alleviation.

20. **C.** Trimethadione is best for petit mal, no help for grand mal. Phenytoin is not absorbed in intramuscular form.

21. **A.** Higher "relative" work loads in normals cause a more pronounced elevation of lactate and creatine kinase. The other statements are true.

22. **D.** It is a persistent quivering, most often of the facial muscles, and at times is seen in polyradiculoneuropathy but more often with multiple sclerosis and brainstem tumors.

23. **E.** Hemorrhage into the right thalamus was added to the other known sites causing unilateral neglect in a recent study; the dorsolateral frontal lobe is also a known site.

24. **B.** Autonomic neuropathy is also common; there is no known effective antidote.

Answers and Comments / 227

25. E. All are correct. Reduced absorption of calcium or changes in parathyroid function may not be necessary for development of bone disease in patients taking phenytoin.

26. B. Sulcal enlargement and ventricular enlargement are common, infarcts and hemorrhages are not infrequent, but subdurals did not occur in this series.

27. C. Male brains weigh about 10% more than female brains on the average. Decline in brain weight begins near age 45.

28. B. The number of selective injections is a marginally significant risk factor, and the presence of arterial stenosis greater than 90% is a strong risk.

29. D. It is usually symmetric (when bilateral), usually involves the globus pallidus, is usually not related to calcium disturbances, and usually does not require further invasive studies.

30. D. The incidence is 12.1/100,000 in Rochester, Minn.; it is more common in males, in older age groups, and with preexisting hypertension.

IV: Infectious Diseases Answers and Comments

1. B. Despite the fact that *C. perfringens* is a frequent isolate from the stools of many normal persons, the establishment of infection with this organism within intra-abdominal abscesses is rare.

2. B. Sporulation of *C. tetani* but not of *C. perfringens* may take place in animal and human tissues. *C. perfringens* will usually form spores only in culture media or the soil.

3. A. *S. aureus* remains the most frequently isolated etiologic agent of endocarditis in heroin addicts.

4. B. All of the parasitic agents listed save *A. lumbricoides* appear to cause infection to a greater degree in patients treated with corticosteroids. The reason ascariasis does not is unclear, as migration from the bowel does occur with *Strongyloides stercoralis*.

5. C. Serum IgG levels are almost invariably markedly elevated in infected myeloma patients. Unfortunately, the IgG is usually nonfunctional.

6. B. Gram-negative infections in leukemia patients appear to be more rapidly fatal than infections with gram-positive organisms.

7. D. Osler's nodes and Janeway lesions are extremely uncommon manifestations of infective endocarditis in the antibiotic era even in the geriatric patient.

8. B. The Jarisch-Herxheimer reaction occurs most commonly following the onset of therapy for syphilis but may occur with any of the disease processes caused by spirochetal organisms, including leptospirosis. The patient may experience transient fever and symptoms of malaise, chills, headache, and myalgia. A transient neutrophilicocytosis occurs at the height of the reaction, which subsides within 24 hours, and its occurrence is not an indication for discontinuance of treatment.

9. C. Few, if any, symptoms of tuberculosis are specific for that disease, and, in fact, this is one of the great mimickers of medicine.

10. C. Orchitis is an extremely unusual manifestation of brucellosis and is usually a complication rather than a presenting symptom. It is seldom seen in the United States.

11. A. The majority of pelvic infections occurring in the presence of indwelling uterine devices may be caused by mixed flora, including a high percentage of anaerobes.

12. D. Streptococcal sepsis is not amenable to therapy with adjunctive steroids.

13. B. Poisoning with *A. phalloides* is predominantly due to the parasympathomimetic alkaloid muscarine resulting in symptoms related to parasympathetic simulation. Muscular tremors, confusion, excitement, and delirium are common in severe poisoning.

14. E. In most cases of gastrointestinal tuberculosis the chest x-ray is entirely negative.

15. D. Large doses of corticosteroids are of little or no therapeutic value in clinical tetanus.

16. B. Proteus OX-K agglutinins (Weil-Felix reaction) are not specific for any particular disease, and rising titers are not diagnostic of Rocky Mountain spotted fever.

17. A. Most patients with juvenile rheumatoid arthritis, whether children or adults, are usually seronegative.

18. E. Although some tetracycline-resistant gonococci have been reported, it is unusual or infrequent in this particular population at the present time. This may now be changing.

19. C. The mortality of *Klebsiella pneumoniae* pneumonia is extremely high, but death usually occurs early rather than late in the course of the illness.

20. B. Surgical intervention is more often necessary than not, since gram-negative osteomyelitis tends to produce significant destruction of bony tissues, necessitating removal of necrotic debris that will perpetuate infection.

21. C. The organisms associated with intrinsic contamination of intravenous fluids are frequently resistant to multiple antimicrobial agents, including cephalothin and ampicillin.

22. B. The pathophysiology differs a great deal between gram-negative and gram-positive bacteremia, the features of each being too extensive to discuss here.

23. E. The incidence of SSPE has not diminished since the introduction of measles vaccine.

24. A. There is no evidence that adenovirus is responsible for a large measure of nosocomially acquired respiratory infections.

25. E. There is no glomerular arteriolitis associated with administration of amphotericin B.

26. D. Although a moderate eosinophilia is often noted in individuals infected by this worm the eosinophilia is not constant and may in fact be absent.

27. C. Amikacin is essentially unbound to serum protein.

28. A. This article by the Center for Disease Control established general guidelines for the prevention of catheter-associated urinary tract infections. It is recommended that once or twice daily perineal care for catheterized patients should include cleansing of the meatal catheter junction with an antiseptic soap, and subsequently antimicrobial ointment might be applied.

29. E. In a study of 1217 children hospitalized with gastroenteritis

Answers and Comments / 231

in Manitoba, Canada, bacterial pathogens were present in 25%. Enterotoxigenic organisms were not of great numerical importance in the etiology of diarrhea in hospitalized children. The etiology of the majority of cases of diarrhea in children remains unknown.

30. E. *Actinomyces* was isolated from four of 13 patients with mandibular osteomyelitis in this series.

31. D. No children with tuberculous meningitis appeared to have normal cerebral spinal fluid findings.

32. C. Adenine arabinoside appears to be a safe and effective agent in the treatment in *herpes simplex* encephalitis. There is little or no evidence of acute drug toxicity due to this compound.

33. E. Many patients with *Y. enterocolitica* infection may present with abdominal symptoms suggestive of appendicitis, but when the appendix is removed, it is usually normal. Some patients have mesenteric lymphomatosis or acute ileitis but not appendicitis.

34. C. There is a statistically significant difference in the duration of symptoms between patients with gonococcal and nongonococcal urethritis. Patients with nongonococcal urethritis usually have symptoms of longer duration than those with gonococcal urethritis ($p<0.0005$).

35. B. All of the patients in this study were shown to have an increased total peripheral eosinophil count.

36. C. This new halophilic *Vibrio* is a pathogen, and most cases (85%) of this disease occur during relatively warm months in men 40 years of age or older. Patients with underlying hepatic disease, particularly hemochromatosis have an unusually high risk of dying after infection with this organism.

37. B. All of the other vibrios listed are halophilic or salt-loving vibrios which have been associated with sea water fish and shellfish as has *Erysiplothrix insidiosa* infection, which may occur after contact of injured skin with fish or shellfish.

38. C. The natural history of sexually acquired chlamydial infection in women has not been defined

39. E. Granuloma inguinale is a chronic indolent and granulomatous disease of the skin and mucous membranes produced by *Calymmatobacterium granulomatis*.

40. E. Self-explanatory

41. C. Of 60 patients with brain abscesses, most presented with signs of an expanding intracranial lesion, and fever was frequently absent. Most brain abscesses originated from otic or paranasal sinus infection, although the majority were of unknown source. In patients with possible brain abscesses, lumbar puncture should be discouraged. Frequently, only minimal information is obtained, and the lethal complication of brain herniation has been repeatedly emphasized.

42. D. Infection with *B. parapertussis* is serologically distinct from infection with *B. pertussis* and there is no cross-immunity.

43. D. There has been a unique case of Whipple's disease in a 54-year-old man with chronic cough and gastrointestinal symptoms in whom the initial diagnosis of Whipple's disease was made by lung biopsy. The bacilliform structures of Whipple's disease were demonstrated in the pulmonary parenchyma of this patient.

44. E. There are trends for more frequent splenectomy in patients with Hodgkin's disease in whom zoster subsequently develops and for more frequent corticosteroid therapy in patients with disseminated zoster. Advanced stages of Hodgkin's disease in itself are not associated with development of zoster and the onset of zoster, does not herald a poor prognosis for the underlying disease. Herpes zoster is thus largely a source of increased morbidity rather than mortality in the population studied and multiple factors appear to predispose to the development of zoster in this group of patients.

45. C. Screening for covert bacteriuria could not be recommended, since a trial involving 208 girls aged 5 to 12 showed that kidney damage associated with infection appears to arise prior to the age of

5 years and that therapy is not effective in preventing further damage.

46. E. A variety of intestinal pathogens have been associated with venereal transmission and symptomatic illness including those listed, with the exception of brucellosis.

47. E. Enterococci are frequently resistant to cefazolin along with the other cephalosporins. Even when the organisms are sensitive, infections do not appear to respond well. Even though there is *in vitro* synergy between cefazolin and gentamicin (with many enterococcal strains), infections respond poorly to this combination.

48. A. The bacteriology in cases of Ludwig's angina usually involves multiple organisms and frequently staphylococci and streptococci are involved. However, gram-negative organisms may be seen including *E. coli* and *Pseudomonas aeruginosa* and anaerobic organisms including *Bacteroides* sps. have also been implicated. Antimicrobial therapy directed at a mixed population is often necessary to the cure of this illness.

49. E. A human reovirus-like agent has emerged as a major etiological agent of acute enteritis of infants and young children in many parts of the world. Although there may be several serologic types responsible for these diseases there are not two different serologic types responsible for disease in infants and in children.

50. E. *Eikenella corrodens*, a facultative anaerobic gram-negative bacillus is surprisingly sensitive to most antibiotics including penicillin, ampicillin, cephalothin, chloramphenicol and erythromycin, gentamicin and vancomycin. However several studies have shown that the organism is resistant to clindamycin and metronidazole.

51. E. In a prospective study of 200 patients, the diagnosis of pseudomembranous colitis was made by proctoscopic examination of the inflamed bowel. The symptoms of fever, abdominal cramps, and diarrhea with or without blood or mucus are not diagnostic or characteristic of pseudomembranous ulcerative colitis.

52. D. Filariform larvae, the result of rhabditiform larvae metamorphosis, may often be seen in stools and are the means of "autoinfection" by penetrating perianal skin.

53. C. Cases of deafness, moderate hearing loss, and vestibular dysfunction were seen in more patients treated with ampicillin than in those treated with chloramphenicol. However, the differences were not statistically significant. The authors emphasized that further research on the therapy of this disease remains to be done.

54. B. There is a low sensitivity and specificity of serologic tests for antipneumocystis antibody, making it difficult to identify potential carriers or individuals with mild to subclinical infections. In a recent outbreak there was epidemiologic and serologic evidence to suggest that acquisition and spread of *Pneumocystis carinii* may have been related to contact with the hospital environment but was insufficient to determine whether spread occurred from patient to staff or staff to patient.

55. B. Primary endocarditis of the right side of the heart is uncommon, usually requiring valvular damage, congenital defects or a left-to-right shunt to nurture a septic process. Secondary right-sided endocarditis is more common and may become the major and persistent focus of pyemia after the inciting cause has been corrected.

56. C. Most congenital cardiac anomalies merit prophylactic antibiotics when patients are to undergo procedures with a high risk of bacteremia. An exception is atrial septal defect, secundum type, where endocarditis is exceedingly rare.

57. A. The presence of obligate anaerobes in mixed infections of intra-abdominal, soft tissue, female genital or oral pulmonary origin was extremely high. Eighty-five percent of aerobic isolates tested were susceptible to either gentamicin or clindamycin and ninety-seven percent of anaerobic isolates were inhibited by clindamycin. A combination of these two agents appeared to be extremely effective empiric therapy despite the life-threatening nature of the infections and the severity of underlying disease.

58. E. Strictly speaking neither *Actinomyces* nor *Nocardia* are fungi but are actually true bacteria and as such are treated with antibacterial antibiotics.

59. E. In this series of 55 patients with candidiasis, 27 of whom that died during candidal infection, 15 were not diagnosed prior to death. Two more patients died while being treated with amphotericin B.

60. A. Hypoxemia may occur in both viral pneumonia as well as in Legionnaires' disease. Viral pneumonias, however, are seldom associated with significant involvement of other major organ systems, and elevated WBC counts are not common.

61. D. Each of the other conditions has been reported as a predisposing factor but no cases of leukemia have been reported as predisposing specifically to staphylococcal sternal osteomyelitis.

62. E. Although it has been theorized that one antibiotic may reduce the toxicity of another, there is no documented evidence at the present time that this actually occurs and/or that combinations can be used in this regard.

63. C. Prophylactic antibiotics have *not* been shown to be effective in reducing the incidence of postoperative infection in patients undergoing exploratory laparotomy.

V: Endocrinology
Answers and Comments

1. B. Pituitary adenomas, usually chromophobe in nature, are probably the most common cause of hypopituitarism occurring in the adult. All of the other diseases listed should be considered in the differential diagnosis.

2. B. The earliest manifestation of pituitary failure in the adult is usually related to decreased gonadotropin secretion. Later findings may relate to hypothyroidism (low TSH), hypoadrenalism (low ACTH), hypoglycemia (low growth hormone and cortisol), or loss of skin pigment (low β-lipotropin and MSH-like pituitary peptides).

3. B. Supraseller extension of the tumor compresses the chaism of the optic nerve, frequently causing bitemporal visual field defects.

4. E. The most specific abnormality in acromegaly is persistent elevation of growth hormone after an oral glucose load. In normal subjects growth hormone is suppressed by glucose.

5. D. The history strongly suggests a hyperprolactinemic state with interference in normal pituitary-gonadal control by a prolactin-secreting pituitary tumor. Such tumors may be too small to cause sellar enlargement, but they are always associated with elevated levels of serum prolactin.

6. C. The abnormal pituitary, which usually contains a small ACTH-secreting adenoma, will suppress with high but not low doses of exogenous glucocorticoids. ACTH secretion is still increased after administration of the adrenal blocking drug, metyrapone, and the hyperplastic adrenals show an exaggerated response to the administration of ACTH.

7. A. Growth hormone and ACTH responses to a hypoglycemic challenge require an intact hypothalamus. Normal secretion of LH and FSH depends upon continuous release from the hypothalamus of a gonadotropin-releasing hormone. Lesions in the hypothalamus frequently cause increased prolactin secretion due to a loss of normal hypothalamic production of a prolactin inhibiting factor.

8. A. The secretion of all the anterior pituitary hormones would be decreased due to direct loss, secondary to infarction, of the hormone-producing cells of the adenohypophysis. Vasopressin secretion would not be impaired because this hormone is synthesized in nerve cell bodies located in the hypothalamus.

9. D. The empty sella is characterized by herniation of the meninges into the pituitary fossa, with enlargement of the sella. Both anterior and posterior pituitary functions are usually preserved.

10. C. TRH stimulates the normal pituitary to secrete both TSH and prolactin. It has no direct action on the thyroid gland.

11. B. Bromocriptine is a long-acting dopaminergic drug capable of suppressing the abnormal secretion of prolactin by certain pituitary tumors. In some patients with growth hormone-secreting tumors (acromegaly), abnormal secretion is also suppressed.

12. B. Growth hormone and ACTH secretion are well-preserved in anorexia nervosa, but gonadotropin secretion is characteristically diminished. Serum T_3 is usually low in anorexia nervosa because of decreased conversion of T_4 to T_3 by peripheral tissues. These defects can usually be corrected by refeeding.

13. C. Items 2 and 4 are the minimum requirements for diagnosis. In some, but not all cases, items 1 and 3 will also be true.

14. B. In contrast to primary adrenal deficiency in which hyponatremia is due to aldosterone deficiency and salt wasting, the hyponatremia of hypopituitarism is usually dilutional and may be attributed to impaired water excretion. The defect is corrected by the administration of glucocorticoids.

238 / Answers and Comments

15. D. The clinical features of inappropriate ADH secretion include hyponatremia and hypo-osmolality of the plasma with inappropriately elevated urine osmolality. Renal function and adrenal cortical function (serum cortisol) are normal. Aldosterone secretion is suppressed and urinary sodium excretion increased due to primary water retention.

16. C. Restriction of water intake will tend to reverse the overexpansion of extracellular fluid volume and will correct the hyponatremia. Attempts to administer salt are of little benefit because the sodium is promptly excreted in the urine. Demeclocycline interferes with the action of vasopressin on the kidney and may be beneficial.

17. C. Angiotensin II is the factor that most directly controls aldosterone secretion. Angiotensin II concentrations are, in turn, controlled by the level of plasma renin activity.

18. D. The patient with primary adrenal insufficiency will already have elevated levels of ACTH and will not respond to exogenous ACTH, no matter how much is given.

19. B. A diagnosis of Cushing's syndrome (cortisol excess) is implied by failure to obtain suppression with a low dose of dexamethasone. A higher dose of dexamethasone will suppress ACTH and cortisol production in most patients with pituitary ACTH excess.

20. E. Adrenal function suppresses normally, ruling out a tumor or Cushing's syndrome. Adrenal androgen overproduction is indicated by the high baseline 17-ketosteroids. A biosynthetic block, either congenital or acquired, is likely.

21. D. Measurement of 24-hour metanephrines, VMA, or catecholamines all give an 80% to 90% diagnostic yield. Repeated measurements increase the yield to over 95%. The other tests listed are less specific, and some, such as the histamine test or adrenal angiography, may precipitate hypertensive crises.

22. A. Stress, diurnal rhythm, and negative feedback by glucocorticoids are the major determinants of ACTH secretion and hence of cortisol secretion.

Answers and Comments / 239

23. B. Pharmacologic doses of glucocorticoids over a prolonged period cause Cushing's syndrome regardless of the type of glucocorticoid used. Pituitary ACTH secretion is suppressed and may be inadequate in the face of stress. Every-other-day administration of steroids can diminish these undesirable effects.

24. E. Almost all adrenal cortical carcinomas show evidence of endocrine function. Unfortunately, the majority prove to be inoperable before they are discovered.

25. E. Abnormalities in aldosterone secretion and renin production may be obvious only after appropriate manipulation of the sodium balance. Not all patients will have frank hypokalemia, but virtually all will have a serum potassium less than 4.0, unless there is K^+ replacement.

26. C. Renal ischemia or acute renal vascular damage can lead to the release of large quantities of renin from the affected kidney(s).

27. B. Metyrapone, which blocks cortisol biosynthesis, will not cause a compensatory elevation of ACTH or of urinary compound S (a 17-hydroxysteroid) in patients with pituitary failure. ACTH, if administered repeatedly, will stimulate adrenal function in such patients, but a single dose often fails to distinguish primary adrenal disease from secondary atrophy.

28. E. Pheochromocytomas can arise in the adrenal medulla or in para-aortic sympathetic tissue. Multiple tumors are common in the familial forms of the disease such as those associated with medullary thyroid carcinoma, von Recklinghausen's neurofibromatosis, or von Hippel-Lindau disease.

29. D. In primary hypothyroidism pituitary TSH secretion will rise before overt hypothyroidism occurs. Thus, the TSH will usually be elevated before circulating levels of T_4 and T_3 fall below the lower limits of the normal range.

30. C. Graves' disease is an autoimmune disorder characterized by the presence of thyroid-stimulating immunoglobulins in the serum.

Antibodies against the TSH receptor on the thyroid-cell membrane can actually mimic the stimulatory effects of TSH.

31. E. Adrenergic-blocking drugs such as propranolol can reduce some peripheral manifestations of thyroid hormone excess without affecting thyroid function. Tachycardia, sweating, and tremor are improved. Propranolol is less likely to cause improvement in longer-term metabolic effects as weight loss or muscle wasting.

32. D. There is a continuous increase in the incidence of hypothyroidism for many years following treatment. Given enough time, the majority of patients treated for Graves' disease are likely to become hypothyroid. The toxic multinodular goiter is more resistant to permanent damage, probably because many areas of the gland will be suppressed at the time of treatment and will not take up the radioisotope.

33. D. The organic iodine administered for the IVP would increase the body iodide pool, dilute the test dose of ^{131}I and reduce the number of ^{131}I counts accumulated by the thyroid. Iodide does not interfere with current methods for measuring circulating thyroid hormones or TSH.

34. B. Estrogens cause increased synthesis of thyroid-binding globulin. Increased circulating TBG causes an increase in available T_3 and T_4 binding sites (reflected by a decreased T_3 resin uptake) and an increase in total circulating T_4. The biologically active free fraction of T_4 would be unchanged.

35. C. TSH is high in primary hypothyroidism and shows an exaggerated response to TRH. In secondary hypothyroidism, TSH is low or normal and shows a diminished response to TRH.

36. B. Administration of exogenous T_4 suppresses the pituitary TSH response to TRH, and endogenous secretion of thyroid hormones ceases. Some of the administered T_4 is converted to T_3 by the liver and other tissues so that measurable levels of serum T_3 are maintained.

37. B. Classic subacute thyroiditis is associated with tenderness although "painless" presentations are now more frequently recognized. In the active stage of the disease, there is release of stored hormone and suppression of iodine uptake by the gland. High antithyroglobulin antibody titres or the development of hypothyroidism would be more consistent with a diagnosis of chronic lymphocytic (Hashimoto's) thyroiditis.

38. D. Previous irradiation to the thyroid is a significant risk factor for the development of thyroid cancer. A nodular goiter or a hyperfunctioning nodule is unlikely to harbor a malignancy. Acute pain and swelling suggests hemorrhage into a preexisting benign nodule or cyst.

39. D. Marked elevation of testosterone with normal adrenal androgen production (17-ketosteroids) suggests a virilizing ovarian tumor. The most common type is arrhenoblastoma, the majority of which are palpable on pelvic examination.

40. D. Addison's disease due to idiopathic or "autoimmune" adrenal failure is often associated with primary ovarian failure, which is presumably also autoimmune in nature.

41. C. The reason for the loss of germ-cell elements is unclear. Lack of spermatogenesis with continuing Leydig cell function leads to elevation in FSH but not LH.

42. D. Amenorrhea with total lack of bleeding after both progesterone and estrogen withdrawal suggests an endometrial abnormality such as uterine synechiae.

43. B. Gradually increasing estrogens in the preovulatory phase are associated with increased pituitary responsiveness to LH-RH (positive feedback). A surge of LH occurs just prior to ovulation.

44. A. The depletion of functioning ovarian follicles leads to reduction in estrogens (particularly estradiol) and progestins and a decreased responsiveness of the ovary to gonadotropins, which are secondarily increased. Estrogen production declines further after the cessation of cyclic ovarian function.

45. C. Testicular size and total plasma testosterone remain normal with advancing age in otherwise healthy males. The free (unbound) fraction of testosterone may decline, however, owing to an increase in testosterone-binding globulin in the plasma. Testosterone secretion and turnover are moderately decreased. Serum LH levels tend to show a gradual increase with age, even when plasma testosterone remains normal.

46. D. Only impotence due to primary testicular disease and associated low serum testosterone is likely to respond to androgen therapy.

47. E. Cholestatic jaundice is associated only with the orally active 17C-alkylated androgens such as methyltestosterone or fluoxymesterone.

48. A. Long-term estogen therapy may cause improved calcium balance and bone mineralization in postmenopausal women.

49. C. These patients have primary hypogonadism characterized by elevated levels of serum gonadotropins. The gynecomastia may be related to a relative increase in the estrogen/testosterone ratio.

50. A. The syndrome may be caused by a variety of lesions of the pituitary or hypothalamus, but in one form (Kallmann's syndrome) there is absence or maldevelopment of the olfactory nerve. In contrast to Klinefelter's syndrome, the male with hypogonadotropic hypogonadism does not have gynecomastia.

51. C. Most testicular tumors are malignant tumors of germ-cell origin (seminomas, embryonal carcinomas, teratomas, or choriocarcinomas). In many germ-cell tumors, there will be elevation of HCG, alpha-fetoprotein, or both markers.

52. E. The ovaries tend to overproduce androgens in the polycystic ovary syndrome. Adrenal androgen production is usually under normal feedback control.

53. D. All occur with increased frequency but symptoms related to nephrolithiasis are probably the most common.

54. E. Gastrectomy leads to decreased absorption of vitamin D and calcium. Clinical osteomalacia may appear years later.

55. A. Only modest supplements of vitamin D should be required, especially if given IM.

56. A. Excess PTH leads to the pathologic findings of osteitis fibrosa cystica in bone, whether the parathyroid hyperfunction is primary or secondary.

57. C. Secondary hyperparathyroidism is found in hypocalcemic states where there is relative resistance to the action of PTH (uremia, intestinal malabsorption). With restoration of normal serum calcium, PTH levels fall to normal.

58. B. Pseudohypoparathyroid patients have normal ability to secrete PTH but show peripheral resistance to the hormone. Large, pharmacologic doses of vitamin D are required to raise the serum calcium in both disorders because of faulty formation of 1,25-OH2D by the kidney.

59. D. Serum chemistries are usually normal in osteoporosis. Decreased bone mass may be detected radiologically only after loss of 30%–50% of the skeletal calcium.

60. A. PTH tends to be elevated secondary to the decreased serum calcium. Serum phosphorus is low.

61. C. Serum alkaline phosphatase is elevated, indicating high bone turnover. Elevated urinary hydroxyproline indicates increased bone resorption. Serum calcium is usually normal, but may become elevated upon immobilization.

62. D. Low fasting glucose with inappropriately elevated serum insulin is the best evidence for insulinoma.

63. C. New vessels lack adequate supporting structures and tend to rupture.

64. E. Tolbutamide and glucagon are both potent stimulants of secretion by insulinomas and have been applied as diagnostic agents.

65. B. The maximal rate of tubular reabsorption for glucose is usually reached at blood levels of 180–200 mg/dl, but some normal individuals have lower thresholds. Conversely, some diabetics, particularly those with renal failure, have higher thresholds. Pentose and fructose react as reducing sugars (Clinitest-positive) but not by the glucose oxidase method for detecting glucose.

66. D. Obese patients are insulin-resistant. They develop diabetes when they cannot adequately increase their insulin secretion to overcome the resistance.

67. E. All of the items listed can cause insulin resistance.

68. A. Human placental lactogen has anti-insulin effects, accounting for increased insulin requirements, especially in the third trimester. Fasting ketogenesis can account for a greater tendency to ketonuria.

69. E. Sorbitol accumulates within the lens of the eye and probably within the brain. When the blood glucose falls, there is a temporary osmotic imbalance causing water to enter the affected tissues.

70. C. Most patients have very low levels of endogenous insulin, but will correct their acidosis with infusion of exogenous insulin at rates of 3 to 10 U/hour. The acidosis is characterized by an increase in unmeasured anions (anion gap) rather than an increase in chloride.

71. A. Some insulin secretion is maintained, and this is apparently enough to prevent rapid lipolysis and ketone-body formation. Blood glucose is generally higher. CNS derangement may be more severe.

72. C. A temporary and paradoxical fall in CSF pH occurs because CO_2 diffuses from the plasma into the brain faster than HCO_3.

73. C. The acidosis is out of proportion to the measurable ketonemia. The unmeasured acid could be β-hydroxybutyrate, a ketone body not measured by the usual nitroprusside test. β-OHB is particularly elevated after alcohol ingestion. Lactic acid might also account for the severity of the acidosis.

74. E. There is a high degree of correlation between diabetic glomerulopathy and retinopathy. Urinary infections and hypertension are treatable contributing factors to renal failure.

75. D. The patient needs more insulin coverage at night, but it is not feasible to increase his morning NPH, since he is already developing hypoglycemic symptoms at the time of peak action. A divided dose is the best solution.

VI: Rheumatology Answers and Comments

1. A. Mycotic infections are rare causes of a destructive granulomatous-type arthritis. Coccidioidomycosis, histoplasmosis, blastomycosis, cryptococcosis, and sporotrichosis, in decreasing frequency, may involve joints in much the same fashion as tuberculosis after hematogenous spread to subchondral bone.

2. B. During the acute phase of Caffey's disease (infantile cortical hyperostosis) the erythrocyte sedimentation rate is often increased and the serum alkaline phosphatase activity is elevated. All other statements are true.

3. A. Diseases characterized as intermittent arthritis syndromes include gout, pseudogout, episodic rheumatoid arthritis, palindromic rheumatism, intermittent hydrarthrosis, familial Mediterranean fever, and Whipple's disease. Rheumatoid arthritis, systemic lupus erythematosus, and rheumatic fever frequently demonstrate remissions and exacerbations but are not usually classified as intermittent arthritis syndromes.

4. E. The inflammatory arteritides include polyarteritis nodosa, hypersensitivity angiitis, rheumatic fever arteritis, allergic granulomatous arteritis, temporal arteritis, rheumatoid arthritis, systemic lupus erythematosus, dermatomyositis, Henoch-Schönlein purpura, and serum sickness. The noninflammatory arteritides include endarteritis obliterans of rheumatoid arthritis and progressive systemic sclerosis, thrombotic thrombocytopenic purpura, and aortic arch syndrome.

5. D. The most frequent reaction to a foreign serum in a previously unsensitized person evolves 7 to 12 days after injection. The onset is acute with variable pruritic, erythematous, and urticarial skin eruptions, together with fever, headache, malaise, edema, nausea vomiting, abdominal pain, and lymphadenopathy. Myalgia, arthralgia, or arthritis may then follow.

6. A. Females are more commonly affected by polymyalgia rheumatica. Constitutional symptoms may be marked and include fatigue, anorexia, weight loss, and fever. A Normochromic normocytic anemia and hyperglobulinemia may be present, but the most obvious laboratory feature is a greatly elevated erythrocyte sedimentation rate. In one-third of cases, polymyalgia rheumatica evolves to a stage that is identical to that of temporal arteritis.

7. C. In de Quervain's tenosynovitis, maximal pain is induced by forced ulnar deviation after the thumb has been placed in the palm of the hand and grasped by the fingers (Finkelstein's sign). Treatment with local injection of steroid and lidocaine usually results in satisfying relief. Activities that might have precipitated tenosynovitis should be avoided. Chronic low-grade symptoms may require splinting at various times.

8. A. Urethritis is the most common clinical feature of Reiter's syndrome and usually presents as a serous sterile urethral discharge with few clinical symptoms.

9. C. Whipple's disease is characterized by fever, abdominal pain, diarrhea, cutaneous hyperpigmentation, adenopathy, and arthritis. Joint symptoms are frequently acute in onset, episodic, and transient, lasting only for several hours or days. Residual joint changes are uncommon.

10. C. Osteoarthrosis classically affects the distal interphalangeal joints of the fingers, the first metacarpophalangeal and carpometacarpal joints of the thumb, the lower part of the cervical spine, the lumbosacral spine, and the large weight-bearing regions, such as the hips, knees, and first metatarsophalangeal joints. This distribution is frequently confirmed by radiographs, which may also reveal the characteristic changes suggestive of the underlying process.

11. E. Rheumatoid factor is seldom seen in juvenile rheumatoid arthritis.

12. D. Soft-tissue rheumatism syndromes are notoriously common and, although only rarely indicative of generalized disease, may be temporarily disabling. They are characterized by sharply localized areas of musculoskeletal pain and tenderness and include such syndromes as tennis elbow, supraspinatous capsulitis, and trochanteric bursitis. Radiographs may reveal some soft-tissue calcification in symptomatic areas, but usually they are completely normal and help confirm the clinical impression that true arthritis is not present.

13. E. All the drugs listed lower serum uric acid. Other drugs that lower the serum uric acid include sulfinpyrazone, allopurinol, salicylates in high doses, and radiocontrast agents.

14. E. The knees are the most frequently involved joints in pseudogout. Other joints may be involved, including the wrists, elbows, shoulders and ankles.

15. E. In children with Lesch-Nyhan syndrome, there is virtually complete deficiency of HG-PRTase. All other characteristics listed are associated with this syndrome.

16. C. Polymyalgia rheumatica is a well-defined syndrome occurring in older individuals and consisting of pain and stiffness in the proximal muscles, accompanied by a very rapid erythrocyte sedimentation rate. Pain and stiffness are noted in the neck and back as well as in the pelvic and shoulder girdles. Morning stiffness is marked. Alpha-2 globulins and fibrinogen may be elevated. Despite the severe pain, findings on examination of the muscles are normal.

17. D. There are no characteristic laboratory findings in intermittent hydrarthrosis. All other statements are true.

18. D. The association of pneumoconiosis and rheumatoid arthritis may give a radiologic picture of multiple, well-defined, hard round shadows scattered throughout both lung fields (Caplan's syndrome).

19. D. Noncartilaginous manifestations of relapsing polychondritis include fever, iritis, episcleritis, cataracts, deafness, aortic insufficiency, and anemia. Death may occur because of tracheal and bronchial collapse and airway obstruction.

20. E. There are no signs of inflammation in affected joints of patients with osteoarthrosis; all other statements are true.

21. A. Sarcoid is associated with variable joint manifestations, which include arthralgias or overt arthritis. Acute or chronic monoarthritis or polyarthritis may be seen. Other clinical evidence of sarcoid, such as fever, skin rash, iritis, and parotid swelling, is frequently present. Hilar adenopathy and a negative tuberculin skin test support the diagnosis.

22. D. The most serious complication of systemic lupus erythematosus is renal involvement.

23. A. Ankylosing spondylitis is characterized by a marked male predominance with onset in the late teens or early twenties; all other statements are true.

24. A. In about 10% of patients with complete agammaglobulinemia, a rheumatoid arthritis–like disease develops, usually in the absence of serum rheumatoid factor.

25. C. In intermittent hydrarthrosis, systemic signs and symptoms are absent. All other statements are true.

26. C. Hypochromic anemia is present in less than one-third of cases of ankylosing spondylitis. Positive tests for rheumatoid factor occur no more frequently than in the general population. The earliest radiologic changes are usually seen in the sacroiliac joints. Eventually the sacroiliac joints become fused, with obliteration of the subchondral margins; the adjacent sclerosis disappears and diffuse rarefaction of the pelvis supervenes.

27. A. Side effects of steroids include skin and muscle atrophy, purpura, osteoporosis, hyperglycemia, diabetes, edema, congestive heart failure, hypertension, hypokalemia, and masking and reactivation of infection (viral, tuberculous, or bacterial). Other side effects are acne, hirsutism, peptic ulcer complications, psychosis, cataract, glaucoma, avascular necrosis of bone, fat redistribution (buffalo hump, moon face), myopathy, menstrual irregularity, and increased calcium excretion and vitamin D antagonism.

250 / Answers and Comments

28. E. The joint pain of palindromic rheumatism may decrease when swelling is maximal. All other statements are true of this disorder.

29. E. Osteogenesis imperfecta is a rare disease that is transmitted by an autosomal dominant gene. Clinically there is severe osteoporosis with multiple fractures that may even occur in utero, blue sclerae, ligamentous laxity, and thinning of the skin. Otosclerotic deafness may occur in later life.

30. B. Pericarditis associated with rheumatoid arthritis is only occasionally symptomatic and only rarely progresses to chronic constricting disease. In rheumatoid arthritis, conservative measures are warranted at the outset of treatment and these are continued as long as indicated. When discussing the nature of the disease with a patient who has had arthritis of a few weeks' to months' duration the prudent physician avoids promises of quick relief or cures and usually refrains from prescribing any antiarthritis medication except aspirin.

31. C. McArdle's disease, a hereditary disorder chracterized by deficiency of muscle phosphorylase, is associated with muscle weakness and pain due to inability of muscle to metabolize glycogen for energy. Characteristically, weakness and cramps develop after a period of muscle activity. In severe cases, chronic weakness is seen. Myoglobinuria is common. Samples of venous blood drawn from the arm during muscle use reveal a decreased production of lactic acid as an end product of glycogen metabolism. Special stains of muscle biopsy specimens reveal excess amounts of glycogen and partial or complete absence of phosphorylase.

32. A. The factors associated with a poor prognosis in rheumatoid arthritis in respect to joint function include persistent disease of more than one year's duration, age below 30 when the patient is first seen by a physician, sustained disease, and the presence of subcutaneous nodules and high titers of rheumatoid factor.

33. C. Epidemiologic studies of osteoarthritis show an increased incidence of local disease in certain occupations when a single joint is exposed to unusual stress, for example the elbow joint in miners and workers using pneumatic drills, the ankle joint in football players, and the hands of cotton workers. Although it is equally common in men and women, severe disease is more common in females. Absence of any constitutional reaction is a *sine qua non* for the diagnosis of uncomplicated osteoarthrosis. In particular, the erythrocyte sedimentation rate should be less than 20 mm/h, the hemoglobin level should be normal, and serologic tests for rheumatoid factor should be negative.

34. A. Joint rest is important in the management of acute monoarthritis due to trauma or internal derangement. Cold applications are advisable in the early stages, both to provide symptomatic relief and to prevent swelling. Warm applications are indicated later to reduce joint swelling. Isometric exercises help to prevent muscle weakness; elastic compression bandages are helpful. Surgical intervention may be indicated if ligamentous or cartilage injury is present.

35. E. Ankylosing spondylitis is an inflammatory disease of adolescents and young adults (especially men) that predominantly affects the large cartilaginous and small synovial joints of the axial skeleton, although peripheral synovial joints may be asymmetrically involved. Thus, the typical pattern of distribution for this arthropathy includes the sacroiliac joints, the intervertebral disk spaces, the apophyseal and costovertebral joints, the symphysis pubis, and the manubriosternal and claviculosternal junctions. In addition, the large synovial joints (especially the hips, knees, and shoulders) may be affected.

36. E. All the tests listed measure the number and function of T cells. Two other valuable tests are lymphocyte response to mitogens, phytohemagglutinin, concanavalin A, or to allogeneic lymphocytes (mixed lymphocyte response); and the production of soluble mediators, such as macrophage inhibitory factor or blastogenic factor.

37. B. Cardiac conduction disturbances, usually first-degree atrioventricular block, occur in about 10% of cases of ankylosing spondylitis. Aortic insufficiency develops in from 1% to 4%. Statements 1 and 3 are true.

38. A. Organized dense fibrous tissue includes tendons, aponeuroses, and ligaments. Unorganized dense fibrous tissue includes fascial membranes, the dermis, periosteum, and organ capsules.

39. C. The crises of sickle cell disease are often associated with intense polyarthralgia, a finding that has been responsible for the mistaken diagnosis of rheumatic fever. On occasion the pain is accompanied by hydrarthroses and other evidence of joint inflammation, which may be the result of small synovial infarctions. All other statements are true.

40. A. Osteitis deformans, or Paget's disease of the bone, is a chronic disorder of the adult skeleton in which the initial destruction and subsequent remodeling leads to enlargement and softening of affected bone. The disease has been found in approximately 1%–3% of persons past age 45, and is most often polyostotic. Familial aggregation has been described and an autosomal-dominant inheritance has been suggested. The bones most commonly affected are the pelvis, femur, skull, tibia, and vertebrae.

41. B. Pachydermoperiostosis is a condition that occurs in young males. There may be a family history. The joints are never swollen or tender, there is no relationship to underlying disease, and the periostosis is usually thicker and denser than in hypertrophic pulmonary osteoarthropathy.

42. E. Most notable among the bone lesions believed to result from sickle cell thrombosis is avascular necrosis of the head of the femur and, less commonly, the head of the humerus, patella, and vertebral bodies. This complication has been encountered in individuals with sickle cell trait, sickle cell C disease, and sickle cell thalassemia, as well as S-S disease.

43. A. Within the first two months of the rheumatic fever attack, at least 80% of patients have an increased antistreptolysin O titer (greater than 200 units in most laboratories, although standards vary). All other statements are true.

44. A. In scalenus anticus syndrome, pressure on the neurovascular bundle may be caused by compression of the bundle between the scalenus anticus muscle and a normal first rib. Hypertrophy and spastic irritability of the muscle are often present. Pain extends from the neck to the hand, usually in an ulnar distribution. Tiredness or weakness of the extremity may follow. Paresthesia and vasomotor disturbances such as Raynaud's phenomenon are common. Applying pressure over the scalenus anticus muscle reproduces symptoms.

45. E. Common manifestations of Behcet's disease are recurrent painful orogenital ulcers and eye inflammation, followed by arthritis, thrombophlebitis, neurologic abnormalities, and skin lesions.

46. B. Clinically the onset of dermatomyositis is gradual, the disease occurs more commonly in females, and there is a peak incidence of the disease in children and again in the fourth to the sixth decade. Vasculitis is prominent in the former, and underlying neoplasia may be present in the cases that occur in later life.

47. E. Patients with "secondary" amyloid often have deposits in kidneys, spleen, liver, and adrenals.

48. C. The anti-inflammatory effects of steroids include: reduced antibody production; impaired cell-mediated immune response; reduction in lymphoid tissue and in circulating eosinophils; and stabilization of lysosomes.

49. A. A number of routine general laboratory tests are helpful and indicated in the diagnosis of patients with rheumatic disorders. Baseline studies should include a white blood cell count and a differential cell count, hematocrit, erythrocyte sedimentation rate, and urinalysis. Leukopenia suggests a diagnosis of systemic lupus erythematosus. The presence of a severe anemia militates against a benign localized disorder, and the patient should be scrupulously studied for serious systemic disease. Similarly, an elevated sedimentation rate is strong evidence for the presence of a more generalized disorder. Abnormal findings on urinalysis favor a diagnosis of systemic lupus erythematosus, vasculitis, or scleroderma rather than rheumatoid arthritis.

50. D. All patients with gout should be instructed in the necessity of continued therapy and a high fluid intake. Alcohol excess, high purine foods, and salicylates should be avoided. Weight reduction should never be precipitous.

VII: Nephrology Answers and Comments

1. B. In alcoholic ketoacidosis, the β-hydroxybutyrate to acetoacetate ratio in plasma is increased.

2. D. The descending limb is water permeable, and the ascending limb is solute permeable.

3. D. The onset of diabetes insipidus is often sudden, whereas that of compulsive polydipsia is likely to be less well defined.

4. D. Chlorpropamide may act in the kidney by inhibiting prostaglandin synthesis.

5. B. In water deprivation, there is contraction of the extracellular fluid and sodium retention.

6. D. The bicarbonate deficit equals 50% of body weight multiplied by the difference between the desired and actual bicarbonate blood level.

7. C. In pure metabolic acidosis, each mmol fall in bicarbonate is associated with a 1.2 mm Hg fall in PCO_2.

8. C. This pattern shows respiratory alkalosis and persistent hyperventilation.

9. C. Salicylates in small doses suppress secretion; in large doses, they suppress both the secretion and reabsorption of urate.

10. A, D. Significant phosphaturia and bicarbonaturia suggest a proximal site of action.

11. A. Thiazides increase magnesium excretion.

12. D. The full natriuretic effect of spironolactone is usually delayed for a few days.

13. C. Specific gravity measures mass and density, not total solute concentration, and protein is less dense than glucose, dextran or dye.

14. D. For each 30°C above 16°C, the specific gravity is 0.001 less than its true value.

15. A. Complement levels are normal in membranous glomerulonephritis.

16. C./17. C./18. D. The initial situation suggested a false-positive test from tolbutamide, but subsequent tests indicate the presence of renal disease, and a biopsy should be done.

19. C. Dysplasias are more diffuse and result in the "string of beads"; poststenotic dilatation reflects the severity of the stenosis.

20. E. Licorice contains a substance with mineralocorticoid activity.

21. D. Urine potassium usually exceeds 30 mEq/24 hr in patients with primary hyperaldosteronism.

22. C. Sar^1-Ala^8 angiotensin is a competitive agonist-antagonist to angiotensin II receptors.

23. B. The mean arterial pressure is 1/3 the difference between the systolic and diastolic pressures added to the diastolic pressure.

24. B. Following chronic licorice ingestion, plasma renin is suppressed because of volume expansion.

25. C. The underlying abnormality is believed to be increased proximal sodium reabsorption.

Answers and Comments / 257

26. B, D. Diuretics stimulate renin release by causing volume contraction.

27. D. Medullary sponge kidney is commonly diagnosed as an incidental finding on workup for urinary symptoms.

28. D. Hypernephroma with invasion of the veins, congestive heart failure, nephrotic syndrome, and often, terminal complications of renal disease which have caused reduction in renal blood flow (e.g., papillary necrosis), may be etiologic causes of renal vein thrombosis.

29. A. If the filtered bicarbonate is lower than the tubular threshold, there will be complete bicarbonate reabsorption.

30. C. Streptococcal infection is followed by acute nephritis after a latent period of 10 days and for rheumatic fever 18 days; the organisms causing these two diseases are serologically distinct.

31. E. In benign essential hematuria (focal glomerulonephritis), hematuria usually develops within a few hours of the onset of the infection.

32. A. C3 levels are low in mesangiocapillary glomerulonephritis.

33. C. This test can detect 5-10 μg/dl proteinuria.

34. C. False precipitation tests occur with tolbutamide and radioopaque dye.

35. C. The patient clearly has orthostatic proteinuria, and elaborate testing is not indicated.

36. D. Penicillamine may cause extramembranous glomerulopathy.

37. B. This course is most consistent with rapidly progressive glomerulonephritis.

38. B. In a controlled trial of relapsing nephrotic syndrome due to minimal lesion, it has been demonstrated that during a steroid-induced remission, cyclophosphamide greatly reduces the probability of relapse when the steroids are withdrawn.

39. A. Micturition and overhydration may reduce the number of bacteria in the urine. There is no relation between IgA and killing of bacteria, but bladder defense is seriously impaired if there is residual urine.

40. A. Leukocyte-containing casts identified in a freshly passed specimen are found in 66% of patients with renal parenchymal infection.

41. B. 60% have *Proteus* organisms.

42. E. These patients frequently present with oliguric acute renal failure.

43. B. Although interstitial infiltration by lymphocytes may occur in glomerulonephritis, the disease affects mainly the glomeruli.

44. A, B. In proximal RTA during severe acidosis, bicarbonaturia disappears, urinary pH decreases appropriately, and acid excretion is not reduced, suggesting that the acidification process of the distal nephron is intact.

45. E. Multiple vacuoles in the tubular epithelium, mainly in the proximal convolutions, are suggestive of hypokalemic nephropathy. Low serum K of short duration may not show these changes.

46. C. This is due to the concentrated acid urine that occurs in people living in the tropics.

47. B. 25-hydrocholecalciferol is converted to 1,25-dihydroxy-cholecalciferol in the kidney.

48. D, E. Magnesium ammonium phosphate stones are found in association with infection with urea-splitting organisms; however, occasionally prolonged excessive use of alkali will result in these stones.

49. B. Retroperitoneal fibrosis may follow the use of methysergide which is used for the prevention of migraine headache.

50. E. The mechanism is unclear but does not appear to be an allergic reaction.

51. E. The association of pulmonary bleeding and glomerulonephritis has been described in all of the listed conditions.

52. D. When osmotic diuretic is ineffective in acute hyperuricemic nephropathy immediate dialysis should be started for removal of uric acid and treatment of uremia.

53. D. With modern dialysis therapy this remains the major complication.

54. B. With progressive renal failure the interval of administration for procainamide should gradually be lengthened to 6, 8 or 12 hours.

55. A. Parathormone levels in uremia are high and cause uremic bone disease.

56. E. When renal function is normal more than two-thirds of an administered dose of carbenicillin is recovered in the urine within 6 hours. The recommended dose in severe renal failure is 2 gm every 12 hours.

57. B. The GFR is increased 40–50% with pregnancy resulting in a low BUN.

58. D. In essential hypertension, unlike preeclampsia, the serum uric acid is normal and the urate to insulin clearance ratio is not decreased.

59. A. Patient A probably has lipoid nephrosis. The other patients may have immune-deposit disease from malaria, secondary syphilis, *Staphylococcus albus* bacteremia and endocarditis, respectively.

60. D. The indications for nephrectomy include tumor, infection, uncontrollable hypertension, and the possibility of recurrence of the original disease.

61. False. It is autosomal recessive.
62. False. It is autosomal dominant.
63. False. The distribution is equal in both sexes.
64. False. About 50% of cases have hypertension.
65. True. Hypertensive cardiac failure is common.

66. A.
67. C.
68. B.
69. D.
70. E.

VIII: Gastroenterology Answers and Comments

1. D. Long-term antacid administration may have significant effects on bone metabolism. The doses required are within the range of those ordinarily administered for the prevention of acid peptic disease during corticosteroid therapy.

2. D. Obstruction is a substantially smaller problem in Crohn's disease of the colon than of the small intestine.

3. B. Though transit seems increased and pancreatic function depressed, stomach emptying has not been shown to be altered by hyperthyroidism.

4. D. Estrogens do effect the liver's excretory capacity in some fashion and are able to produce hepatic adenomas. An excess of pigment stones has not been noted.

5. D. A toxin apparently produced by *Clostridia* seems to be responsible for the cytotoxicity in pseudomembranous enterocolitis following antibiotic administration. The antibiotics permit overgrowth of the *Clostridia*.

6. C. In a large study performed in Denmark, combined gastric and duodenal ulcer was identified as the most significant negative prognostic indicator for survival. Diagnosis under age 50 was not associated with an excessive number of deaths.

7. D. Outpatient liver biopsy has been reported in several large studies and would seem to be a safe, cost-effective procedure if precautions permitting adequate selection and post-biopsy observation of patients are carefully followed.

8. B. The Veteran's Administration study of the use of hepatitis B immune globulin after needle stick exposures suggested that two doses of specific immune globulin were significantly better in attenuating or preventing the development of hepatitis B than was the treatment with immune serum globulin of the conventional variety. It should be noted that this represents a relatively low volume inoculum, and these results may not be applicable to transfusion infections.

9. E. Although the success rate of nonoperative therapy is only in the range of 50%, it seems the most appropriate first step in the treatment of this complication of pancreatitis.

10. E. Though all have shown promise, when carefully studied none of the measures mentioned can be shown to statistically improve the treatment of pancreatitis. Generally putting the pancreas at rest is still the approach employed.

11. D. CEA assays when positive do not completely correspond to positive diagnosis by cytology; thus, the two examinations taken together will identify more malignant effusions than either used alone.

12. B. In one large series, low levels were found in white children only after age 5. Low levels were found in black children after age 3.

13. C. It seems increasingly evident that alcoholics who develop liver disease have some distinguishing feature or factors that render them more susceptible to liver damage.

14. C. In at least one large study the level of the serum bilirubin seemed to be the best indicator of progression of the disease and had the closest correlation with the length of survival for the patient.

15. E. The development of edema, usually secondary to or in combination with a high sodium content and rapid administration, is the most common complication, followed by diarrhea and hyperglycemia. Mechanical difficulties and congestive heart failure are substantially less frequent.

16. D. Only in livers damaged by nonalcoholic disease is hepatocellular carcinoma associated with evidence of hepatitis B infection in this country.

17. E. Flat villi in small intestine biopsies are not diagnostic of any specific disease, though they do remarkably narrow the differential diagnosis.

18. D. Acute doses of alcohol will increase pancreatic secretion, though obviously, chronic doses producing pancreatitis may result in its decrease. Response of splanchnic circulation is variable.

19. E. A wide variety of neuromuscular diseases can give rise to upper esophageal sphincter dysfunction.

20. C. In one large series, the often-mentioned appearance of right chest findings with amoebic liver abscess were found to occur in less than half of the patients studied.

21. D. The most common association seems to be between the ingestion of thiazide diuretics and the development of acute pancreatitis.

22. C. Broad-spectrum antibiotics that can suppress the growth of enterotoxigenic *E. coli* have been found effective in preventing travelers' diarrhea.

23. B. While all of these are probably factors in nutritional deficiencies occurring in liver disease, failure of dietary intake remains the most common problem. The other factors, however, should not be overlooked.

24. A. Recent studies show a change from earlier figures when terminal ileal disease seemed to predominate. At present, ileocolic disease represents the most common presentation.

25. C. In at least one study, ultrasonic cholangiography was found to be most sensitive in those individuals who had established fairly long-standing extrahepatic obstruction. It has a relatively low sensitivity early in the disease, i.e., when the bilirubin is below 10 mg/dl.

26. E. While all of these may be factors in the development of cancer in association with chronic ulcerative colitis, the most constant association seems to be the presence of dysplasias in the colonic epithelium.

27. A. Diabetes mellitus is far less common in young people with idiopathic hemochromatosis (34% frequency as opposed to 82% frequency in older patients). The other mentioned complications seem to occur in almost the same frequency in both the young and old.

28. E. While the mechanisms are multifactorial, each of the nutrients listed probably is affected by bacterial overgrowth syndromes.

29. C. One recent study showed highly significant success rate for the use of H_2 blocking agents in treating anastomotic ulcers. A great deal of evaluation remains to be done to firmly establish this assay as the therapy of choice in this difficult problem.

30. E. Steatorrhea is not likely to occur unless there is also impairment of bile acid secretion.

31. A. While other hormones may affect the gallbladder, in physiologic circumstances, cholecystokinin is probably the only effective hormone.

32. A. A study of lactase-deficient American Indians suggest that they usually can tolerate at least a glass of milk a day (18 grams of lactose) without symptoms. Total abstinence from milk products is often unnecessary in treating lactose deficiency.

33. D. Once cirrhotic portal hypertension is established, abstinence from drinking apparently has little effect on significant morbidity factors such as encephalopathy, bleeding, and ascites.

34. A. Randomized studies that support the use of steroids are slowly beginning to appear in the literature. Though admittedly not all studies have been able to show that this effect is statistically superior to no therapy at all.

35. E. While the esophagus may clearly be acid sensitive, it may also be sensitive to a variety of foods in the absence of titratable acidity.

36. E. Apparently the esophagus responds to infusion of any volume with a contraction of the upper esophageal sphincter, which presumably keeps us from choking.

37. C. In one large evaluation of patients in this category, significant lesions were found in 41.5% of the patients. Eleven percent of the patients had carcinoma, and 6.5% had cecal telangiectasia.

38. A. In studies directed toward evaluating the need for fiber in the diet, correlations of this sort would tend to support the effect of fiber on these seemingly disparate diseases.

39. A. While psychiatric symptoms are common, the ultimate evaluation is more often that of neurologic disease rather than psychiatric disease. Hepatic presentations are more common in childhood, and hemolytic anemia and bone disease are the least common presentations.

40. A. At least one half of the patients remain free of symptoms. The complications associated with definitive procedures at the time of emergency operation are such that the policy of deferring definitive procedures until a later difficulty develops seems most appropriate.

41. D. Alcoholic cirrhosis is involved as a risk factor in the development of pigment stones. It has not been established as having a role in the development of cholesterol gallstones.

42. C. While the incubation period for clinical illness may be a period of months, sensitive radioaminoassays show the presence of surface antigen in the circulation very promptly after exposure.

43. C. While the statement is often made that alcoholism leads either to pancreatitis or liver disease, there is considerable overlap of individuals with involvement of both organs.

44. E. The factor causing the pulmonary edema is not clear, but it does not seem to be related to the more usual pathways for development of pulmonary edema.

45. C. While the final word is probably not in, several prospective studies showed a highly significant degree of protection against recurrence of peptic ulcer with minimal side effects from the use of long-term maintenance therapy with cimetidine.

46. D. In one study, from England, of a substantial number of patients the spread of inflammation even in severe disease was limited to 30% of the patients. Operative intervention was required in only one-third of the patients, and the cancer risk in that ten-year interval was identified as small.

47. D. While chenodeoxycholic acid will elevate the transaminases, ursodeoxycholic acid will not. Other laboratory tests of liver function do not appear to be affected.

48. C. Both ursodeoxycholic and chenodoxycholic acid have been found to be effective in dissolving gallstones, thought the parameters most appropriate for their application remain to be fully elicudated.

49. E. While most non-cholera *Vibrio* infections are associated with shellfish and salt-water exposure, other sources including contaminated well water, cold asparagus, and egg salad have been reported.

50. E. All sorts of nutritional deficiencies not only of calories but of trace compounds and administered medications have been described with intestinal bypass. Metabolic disorders such as deranged oxalate metabolism may produce additional extraintestinal manifestations.

51. C. With alcohol intoxication, responses of the smooth muscle in the esophagus seem less vigorous.

Answers and Comments / 267

52. A. Once again another study has shown that it seems clear that steroids do not offer much in the long-term control of Crohn's disease.

53. A. Allogeneic bone marrow transplantation is added to the list of etiologies for veno-occlusive disease. It has been thought but not proved to be related to graft-versus-host reactions.

54. B. Apparently the larger you are the slower your stomach empties when dealing with solid food.

55. E. All of these plus an impressive list of additional secondary causes for intestinal pseudo-obstruction have been described.

56. B. The addition of cholecystectomy to vagotomy and pyloroplasty seems to result in diarrhea secondary to a change in the handling of bile acids. This will respond to bile-acid binding.

57. E. The mechanisms were unknown but all of these features have been regularly associated with polyposis coli in Peutz-Jeghers syndrome.

58. E. Endoscopy is considered important, since secondary forms of achalasia may occur in individuals with carcinoma, particularly of the stomach. This secondary sort of achalasia may have all of the clinical, radiographic, and manometric features of the primary achalasia.

59. E. *Giardia* seems to produce derangement of brush border activities, which, following eradication, can usually be expected to improve.

60. B. Not only transient levels in hepatocellular enzymes but also unconjugated hyperbilirubinemia have been reported with the use of chenodoxycholic acid.

61. C. Not only have arthritis, glomerulonephritis, and arteritis been associated with the presence of circulating immune complexes incorporating hepatitis B surface antigen, but also the occurrence of prodromal urticaria has been related to the deposition of immune complexes in the skin.

62. E. Multiple factors probably give rise to thrombocytopenia including folate deficiency, marrow depression, and a degree of hypersplenism.

63. E. While generally both the skin and the jejunal lesion if present will improve, this is not invariable and all combinations have been observed.

64. B. In at least one study the patients' sex, smoking habits, and alcohol consumption had little to do with the development of recurrence of gastric ulcer in a four-year interval.

65. B. Only long-term glucocorticoid administration or Cushing's disease will raise the serum gastrin in a significant fashion.

66. E. In at least one large kindred with familial visceral myopathy, specimens at all levels of the intestinal tract and the urinary bladder showed changes in the smooth muscle.

67. E. Endocrine tumors of the pancreas have not only been found to secrete all of the hormones listed, but tumors secreting vasoactive intestinal peptide (VIP) and some tumors secreting multiple hormones have also been described.

68. E. Diabetic enteropathy can produce diarrhea secondary to enteropathy in the small bowel and constipation when the large bowel is primarily affected.

69. A. In one large study over half of the adenomatous polyps found were greater than 1 cm in diameter, and most were on the left side of the colon. In this study well over half the patients had only a single adenoma.

70. D. Pancreatin alone does as well as pancreatin with either an antacid or enteric coating. Careful studies have shown reduction of steatorrhea with the addition of cimetidine.

71. A. While ampicillin can cause pseudomembranous enterocolitis, it also can present as an allergic reaction with bloody diarrhea and without evidence of pseudomembranous disease. Several studies suggest that this might be a more common presentation.

72. C. Cimetidine seems to have basically an antacid effect and does not affect either positive Bernstein tests or healing of the mucosa in individuals with esophageal reflux.

73. E. Biliary tract dysfunction that responds to therapy with antigiardial drugs has frequently been described most often by nonvisualization at cholecystography.

74. D. Muscle appears normal, but the number of ganglion cells seem remarkably reduced in the esophagus of elderly patients.

75. A. Those compounds that seem to inhibit secretion rather than just neutralize acid seem to halt gastric protein loss.

IX: Pulmonary Answers and Comments

1. A. The antibiotic regimen should be streptomycin and chloramphenicol. The ulcer and pericarditis should suggest tularemia.

2. B. The etiological agent is varicella virus. Varicella pneumonia occurs at the onset of chickenpox.

3. A, B, C, D. The diagnosis of infection with *A. fumigatus* depends upon: repeated cultures of the organism from the trachea, a positive serum precipitin reaction for *A. fumigatus*, and an immediate (type I) or delayed (type III) skin reaction to aspergillus antigen.

4. C. *Toxocara canis* is the parasite responsible for the visceral larva migrans seen in this patient.

5. F. *Staphylococcus aureus* is the most common pathogen isolated from patients with cystic fibrosis. *Pseudomonas aeruginosa* is also frequently isolated.

6. B, C. Knife grinding and gold mining are occupations in which there is an increased risk of tuberculosis because in both trades there is an appreciable exposure to silica.

7. D. The isolation of atypical bacilli is frequent in dust diseases, in particular silicosis.

8. B, E. *M. phlei* and *M. fortuitum* are the bacillus because they are rapid growers, whereas the other bacillus are slow growers.

9. A, C, D, E. PAS and streptomycin, streptomycin and viomycin, pyrazinamide and PAS, and viomycin and INH should be avoided in the treatment of tuberculosis. Streptomycin and viomycin both have toxic effects on the eighth nerve, and pyrazinamide and PAS, and, PAS and ethionamide are hepatotoxic.

10. C. Thoracotomy and removal of the right middle lobe should be the next step in this case because despite the positive skin tests, the lesion has about a 40% chance of being a carcinoma. Resection, therefore, is the most appropriate therapy.

11. A, B. Paralysis of a vocal cord and diaphragmatic paralysis due to an upper lobe tumor are both contraindications to surgery in lung cancer. Unless it is bloodstained, pleural effusion is not necessarily a contraindication.

12. B, D. Left recurrent laryngeal paralysis and paralysis of the diaphragm by a lesion situated just above the left hilum are complications of lung cancer that indicate inoperability. Complete blockage of the left pulmonary artery renders resectability unlikely, but is not an absolute contraindication as it is when the right pulmonary artery is completely occluded. Pleural effusion may be secondary to atelectasis and pneumonia, rather than an extension of the tumor to the pleura.

13. B, C. Superior vena cava obstruction and the presence of palpable nodes in either supraclavicular fossa are both circumstances under which a biopsy of scalene nodes, in suspected lung cancer, would yield a positive diagnosis. Nonpalpable supraclavicular nodes yield a positive diagnosis in only 5-10% of patients undergoing biopsy. When there is superior vena cava obstruction, biopsy should be done with caution because of the risk of bleeding due to increased venous pressure.

14. D. Instillation of nitrogen mustard into the pleural space is the treatment of choice in this case. Radioactive gold was used in the past, but is more expensive, presents a problem in regard to radiation, and is more likely to lead to localized tissue damage when the fluid is loculated.

15. D. Special radiographic views to show upper right ribs and vertebrae would be helpful in this case because the symptoms suggest a thoracis inlet tumor, which is peripherally situated and often very small. Characteristically it causes rib erosion.

16. A. Chemotherapy is beneficial in lung cancer if there is superior vena cava obstruction. The preferred treatment of choice in vertebral metastases is radiotherapy.

17. C. Adrenal carcinoma is the probable diagnosis in this case. The metyrapone test does not elevate the serum cortisol in the ectopic ACTH.

18. C. A serum calcium test is likely to confirm the suspected diagnosis in this case because the peripheral rounded shadow suggests a squamous carcinoma. This histological type is most commonly associated with the secretion of parathormone.

19. A, C, E. Serum sodium 112 mEq/l, urinary sodium in 24 hours 170 mEq/l, and simultaneous demonstration of a plasma osmolality of 250 mOsm/kg and a urine osmolality of 650 mOsm/kg might be present in this case. The development of confusion and semicoma after drinking water suggests that he has inappropriate secretion of ADH.

20. B, C, D, E. The association of clubbing and hypertrophic pulmonary osteoarthropathy is most frequently seen in pulmonary or pleural malignancy. It is less commonly seen in pulmonary intrathoracic tumors, such as fibromas. It is also seen in pyogenic lung abscess.

21. A, D, E. Resection of the tumor, vagotomy when resection is not possible, and thoracotomy without resection have been accompanied by remissions in the pulmonary osteoarthropathy. In some unresectable tumors, radiation therapy has been beneficial. Hormones are of no help.

22. D. A mass present in pure red cell aplasia is likely to be located in the anterior mediastinum. Red cell aplasia is sometimes associated with the presence of a thymoma.

23. C. Although the lesions could be a metastatic disease, the fact that he has been treated with steroids and other chemotherapeutic agents, makes secondary fungal infection more likely.

24. A, E. Bauxite and Cadmium may produce pulmonary emphysema. Bauxite leads to "traction emphysema" from adjacent fibrotic scarring.

25. B, C, D, E. Progressive massive fibrosis may be found in hematite miners' lung, kaolin lung, asbestosis, and graphite lung. Massive shadows are rare in asbestosis but they can occur.

26. B, E. Berylliosis is a progressive disease. Hilar adenopathy occurs in both sarcoidosis and berylliosis but is smaller in size in the latter. When symptomatic, berylliosis is associated with lung disease but not with hilar involvement free of parenchymal nodularity. Tuberculin sensitivity is unaffected by berylliosis. Beryllium is ubiquitous and frequently found in lung tissue in the absence of granulomatous disease.

27. A, D. Focal emphysema is frequently seen surrounding the coal macule in simple coal workers' pneumoconiosis. The initial evidence that coal dust inhalation could result in pneumoconiosis was reported in coal trimmers at the Cardiff docks. These men were handling coal washed free of silica. Symptoms of dyspnea are far more likely to occur in miners who have chronic bronchitis or emphysema. Spirometic abnormalities correlate better with a smoking history than with coal dust exposure. Several early studies suggested an association of CWP with tuberculosis. This has been disproved by more extensive and more recent studies.

28. D. The association of peripheral nodules (0.5 to 5.0 cm) in coal miners with rheumatoid arthritis was first reported by Caplan in 1953. Most of these miners have rheumatoid factor in their serum. The presence of rheumatoid factor in this clinical setting is very strong circumstantial evidence for this syndrome.

29. D. The ubiquitous presence of asbestos production in building materials (viz. insulation, roofing, flooring compounds, pipe lagging, etc.) make a demolition worker particularly prone to asbestosis. The physical findings and chest x-ray findings, particularly the diaphragmatic pleural plaquing, confirm the diagnosis of asbestosis. Pleural plaquing is not seen in silicosis, Shaver's disease (Bauxite lung) or idiopathic interstitial fibrosis. Mesotheliomata are more likely to occur in asbestos workders, but the x-ray did not show a density suggestive of a tumor.

30. A, B, E. Silica is being used in certain forms of enameling and abrasive soap manufacturing. Mining in general involves clearing silicaceous overburdens. Iron oxide is used as silver polish. Corundum smelting involves exposure to Al_2O_3.

31. B. Disodium cromoglycate has no bronchodilating effect. It works by preventing the release of bronchoconstrictor mediators from mast cells. It cannot be taken orally or by injection.

32. A, B, C, D. The patient with "pure emphysema" occupies one end of the spectrum of chronic obstructive lung disease. Nicknamed "pink puffers", these patients have progressive, severe dyspnea and marked airway obstruction with little sputum production. They seem able to maintain adequate PaO_2 levels, often with evidence of hyperventilation, until close to death. $PaCO_2$ is frequently normal, occasionally low, but rarely high except in the late stage of this disease. The heart appears small radiographically. Dilated proximal arteries are frequently seen with marked vascular attenuation in central and peripheral lung fields. Cor pulmonale occurs infrequently except late in the course of the disease.

33. C. Destruction of alveolar walls is found in panacinar emphysema. The definition of emphysema (Ciba Symposium) is "a condition of the lung characterized by increase beyond the normal in the size of air spaces distal to the terminal branchiole, either from dilatation or from destruction of their wall." The ATS definition requires disruption of the alveolocapillary surface.

34. A. Right upper lobe bullous disease is the correct diagnosis in this case. Deviation of the trachea to the right would occur with a collapse of the right upper lobe. Cavitation would not cause hyperresonance and overinflation. Pleural effusion on the right would present in dullness on the right. Macleod's syndrome would not result in tracheal deviation to the left.

35. A, B, D. In the management of "shock lung" (ARDS), institution of positive end expiratory pressure (PEEP) may result in pneumothorax, reduced cardiac output and pneumomediastinum. Oxygen toxicity may be avoided by use of PEEP. By reducing ventilation to perfusion mismatching, oxygen levels in arterial blood rise sufficiently to reduce the FIO_2 to less than toxic levels. Gastric dilatation should not occur unless the endotracheal tube is incorrectly placed.

36. B, D, E. Respiratory alkalosis, hypocalcemia, and hypomagnesemia may result in this case. Tetany results when the membranes of nerve cells become increasingly permeable to Ha^+ ion, due to changes in extracellular fluid ionic levels. Tetany also results when Ca^{++} ion, Mg^{++} ion, or H^+ ion are reduced in concentration. Hypokalemia exerts a protective effect against tetany due to reduced Ca^{++} ion concentration.

37. B, C, D. Allergy to iodine is a contraindication to lung scanning using macroaggregated human albumin. In a patient with contraction of the pulmonary vascular bed, large particles may be dangerous.

38. C, D. Serum cholesterol, free fatty acids, and total lipids dropped after the use of hypertonic glucose. Apparently, this works to reduce the mobilization of stored fat, thus reducing the incidence of clinically recognized fat emboli. Corticosteroids have been shown to decrease the toxic effects of fatty acids on lung tissue.

39. C, D. Attempts to detect iliac vein thrombosis with ^{131}I fibrinogen yield little information because background radiation is high enough to mask thrombosis. The Doppler technique is also ineffective in detecting iliac thrombosis. Venography is the most useful technique although physical examination is sometimes helpful.

40. A. Muscle manipulation, electrical stimulation and heparin seem more effective when applied during surgery.

41. A, C. Amphotericin B must be given in dextrose solution because it precipitates in saline. Its major toxicity is renal, but this is not increased by concurrent use of 5-fluorocytosine. Heparin can be used to reduce incidence of phlebitis. Total dose for most systemic fungal infections is not known, but a minimum of two grams is not considered adequate.

42. A, C. Various studies of asthmatics have shown a 1-5% allergenicity to asthma. Nasal polyposis is common in this group.

43. B, D, E. In an acute attack of pancreatitis, elevated glucose and glucagon levels have been observed. Calcium, sodium, and potassium are observed to drop to lower than normal levels in an acute attack. The elevated glucagon levels are believed to be related to the glucose intolerance demonstrated by these patients. Pleural effusions, believed to be transported from peritoneal cavity, are seen in about 55% of cases. These exudates are frequently bloody and have high amylase levels.

44. B. Bronchoscopy is indicated in this case.

45. C. Pneumothorax is present in 1-2% of newborns. Although one-third are normal newborns, two-thirds had hyaline membrane disease and many of these required mechanical ventilation (Arch. Dis. Child. 50:449, 1975). This occurrence is believed due to vigorous inspiratory effort, frequently transiently reaching 100 cm of negative intrathoracic pressure.

46. A. Although PVC polymers thermally degrade to chlorine, phosgene, HCl, and many other organic substances, HCl is the major toxic product. It causes irritation to the mucous linings at concentrations of 15 ppm, but is considered to reach the alveoli adsorbed from soot particles. The onset of symptoms is usually delayed by 1-6 hours. Mucosal irritation may not be appreciated if sufficient carbon monoxide has been inhaled to reduce mental function.

47. C. Acute noncardiac pulmonary edema due to CH_2Cl_2 is the main hazard of the inhalation of methylene chloride (CH_2Cl_2) paint removers. However, methylene chloride is rapidly metabolized to carbon monoxide and can have toxic effects by this means. Since it is absorbed by fat stores, the COHb level can be expected to remain elevated if the exposure is long or fairly intense.

48. A, B, D, E. Microscopically, the lungs might be expected to show histiocytic cellular infiltration, foamy macrophages, plasma cell infiltration and proteinaceous deposits in alveoli. The clinical data describes what used to be referred to as "Hand-Schüller-Christian syndrome" but is now believed best termed eosinophilic granuloma. All of the stated microscopic findings may be present at varying stages of this disease except fibroblastic proliferation.

49. C. Most pickwickian patients hypoventilate but have no evidence of airway obstructions.

50. A, B, C, E. The usual aspergilloma is a fungus ball within a cavity. The other diseases result in cavitation by differing mechanisms. In coal worker's pneumoconiosis complicated (or P.M.F.) there is evacuation of a liquid center. In klebsiella, lung necrosis results in cavity formation. The lesion of Wegener's causes necrosis of lung tissue. In pulmonary embolism, infection distal to infarction can cause cavitation, as can ischemic necrosis.

51. A, D, E. Acute pulmonary edema can result if a large quantity of pleural effusion is evacuated too rapidly; removal of up to 600 ml is considered safe. The inhalation of phosgene or ozone can result in acute pulmonary edema. Phosgene-caused pulmonary edema may be delayed for many hours. Ozone concentration, as little as 9 ppm, can cause edema. Pulmonary fibrosis and alveolar proteinosis may result in congestive heart failure when pulmonary insufficiency becomes severe.

52. C, D. Immediate relief of dyspnea can be accomplished by thoracentesis. Each cubic centimeter of fluid removed allows a similar increase in vital capacity. Since the tumor is likely to be radiosensitive, a course of mediastinal radiation should be undertaken to relieve lymphatic obstruction. Chemotherapy is also effective.

53. A, B, D. Hypertrophic pulmonary osteoarthropathy is most often associated with carcinoma of the bronchus. It is also seen in pleural fibroma, pulmonary sepsis and aortic aneurysm. Resection of the tumor, thoracotomy without removal of tumor and resection of vagus nerves has resulted in regression of this process. Serum growth hormone has been reported to be elevated in some, but not all series.

54. C. Conjunctival biopsy would be most productive in this case because the noncaseating granuloma suggests sarcoidosis.

55. B, C, E. Gram stain of sputum may show typical gram-positive diplococci, yet *Staphylococcus aureus* or normal oral flora may be frequently cultured. The smear is an indication of the organism but it is not diagnostic. With special typing serum, a swelling of the bacteria capsule (quellung) can be demonstrated in sputum or cultured pneumococci. Dimpling of the culture of pneumococci occurs at 48 hours.

X: Oncology
Answers and Comments

1 C. Studies have shown that nodular poorly differentiated lymphocytic lymphomas and nodular well-differentiated lymphocytic lymphomas did not require treatment for an average of 32 months and 8 or more years, respectively.

2. A. Studies show that combination combination chemotherapy increases complete remission, increases total percentage of objective responses and is generally more toxic. In the few randomized studies done, chemotherapy has not been demonstrated to increase life expectancy.

3. C. Tamoxifen (ICI 46474) is an oral antiestrogen that is very useful in ER+ metastatic disease. Although active in premenopausal disease, because of the side effects from the high doses required, it is used almost exclusively in the postmenopausal group.

4. A. Estrogen receptor positive breast cancers are more common in the menopause. Such tumors usually respond to hormonal manipulation.

5. D. In most human cancers, adjunctive therapy has not been helpful in increasing cures. The most convincing data is in premenopausal breast cancer and Wilms' tumor, with suggestive data in osteogenic sarcoma.

6. C. Histiocytic lymphoma involves the marrow initially in less than 10%, can be cured with multiagent chemotherapy, such as BACOP or CHOP bleomycin, and is rarely nodular. Recent studies subclassifying it have shown a better prognosis if the histiocytic lymphoma is the large, cleaved type.

7. E. Immunoblastic lymphadenopathy appears to be a nonneoplastic hyperimmune proliferation triggered by a hypersensitivity reaction.

8. A. The main drawback of *cis*-diaminodichloroplatinum is nausea and emesis; liver toxicity is rare; bone marrow; renal and otic are usually manageable. It is eliminated through the kidney.

9. A. Oat cell carcinoma has been shown to be usually disseminated at the time of diagnosis, precluding effective surgery. It responds well to chemotherapy and radiation.

10. A. The pathologic classification of melanoma according to Clark's levels or Breslow's thickness affords a quantitation of the risk of regional node involvement which is greater than 50% in the examples shown.

11. C. A control prospective trial has demonstrated that BCG treatment will delay recurrence but not increase cure rate of primary malignant melanoma. Unfortunately, systemic illness with BCG will occasionally require antitubercular therapy.

12. A. The three agents that have some activity in primary brain tumors are: VM-26 (podophyllotoxin), procarbazine and BCNU (nitrosourea), particularly the latter two.

13. E. Mithramycin allegedly interferes with osteoclast function; oral phosphosoda leads to the exceeding of calcium's solubility in the blood; calcitonin inhibits bone resorption and Indocin inhibits prostaglandin mediated hypercalcemia.

14. E. Pericardial effusion and transverse myelitis are complications primarily of radiation, whereas acute leukemia and prolonged myelosuppression are more commonly caused by the combination of radiation and chemotherapy.

15. B. The nitrosoureas are the most recent agents demonstrating renal injury.

16. A. In the treatment of metastatic carcinoma of the kidney,

CCNU (vinblastine) has recently been reported to produce good responses, and specific and nonspecific immunotherapy has produced a surprising 25% response.

17. C. Although quite toxic, the combination of *cis*-diaminodichloroplatinum, bleomycin and vinblastine, is highly effective and leads to an appreciable number of cures.

18. A. Hepatic adenomas develop from the use of oral contraceptives but regress when these chemicals are withdrawn. Angiosarcomas develop in vinyl chloride workers.

19. C. Studies in preoperative radiation have shown a definite, though small, increase in disease-free state and a decrease in local recurrence in carcinoma of the rectum.

20. C. A family has been found where all cases had this disease.

21. D. Hexamethylmelamine in combination with cytoxan, methotrexate and fluorouracil has produced very good results, in treatment of ovarian carcinoma.

22. A. DTIC is useful in neural crest tumors, like melanoma, and now apparently it is useful in the treatment of the malignant carcinoid syndrome.

23. C. It is only recently that the importance of diaphragmatic metastases at initial staging surgery has been recognized.

24. E. A recent study documented a 63% objective response rate for the use of *cis*-diaminodichloroplatinum, methotrexate and bleomycin in the treatment of head and neck tumors.

25. E. Unfortunately, no combination of agents is clearly superior to FU alone.

Dear Doctor

Should you wish additional samples of any of the Stuart Pharmaceuticals products listed below, please have your Nurse contact me at:

Stuart Representative Card

☐ **MYLANTA**®
☐ **MYLANTA**-**II**®
☐ **AlternaGEL**™

☐ **MYLICON**-**80**®

☐ **SORBITRATE**®
ISOSORBIDE DINITRATE

☐ **DIALOSE**®**PLUS**
☐ **KASOF**®
☐ **EFFERSYLLIUM**®

☐ **STUARTINIC**®
☐ **FERANCEE**®-**HP**